ADOLESCENT LIVES   3

A SERIES EDITED BY JEANNE BROOKS-GUNN

The New Gay Teenager

RITCH C. SAVIN-WILLIAMS

HARVARD UNIVERSITY PRESS

Cambridge, Massachussetts
London, England
2005

Library of Congress Cataloging-in-Publication Data

Savin-Williams, Ritch C.
The new gay teenager / Ritch C. Savin-Williams.
p. cm. — (Adolescent lives ; 3)
Includes bibliographical references and index.
ISBN 0-674-01673-4
1. Gay teenagers—Social conditions. 2. Gay teenagers—Psychology.
3. Gay teenagers—Mental health. I. Title. II. Series.
HQ76.25.S395 2005   2004059787

To my friend, Lisa Diamond

Contents

Preface

When I began my first survey research with same-sex-attracted adolescents and young adults in 1983 and taught my first "gay-related" college course in 1984, now titled "Gender and Sexual Minorities," my actions grew out of needs both personal and professional. The personal needs I gradually resolved—I named my sexual/romantic attractions, involved myself as an active member of various gay communities, became a part-time therapist specializing in gay issues, and gained a partner who enriched my life.

The professional development has evolved more slowly, but now at last I can hope that contemporary teenagers are bringing the sexual identity era to a close. Gay people have historically too readily accepted the inevitability and desirability of divisions based on sexual categories. It's not that same-sex attractions are disappearing—indeed, they appear to be on the upswing as young people more freely share with each other their same-sex feelings. They're not embarrassed by gayness, don't consider it deviant, and see it all around them—on television, in movies, in songs, in cultural icons, among their friends.

I celebrate this development, because my lifetime professional dream—that homosexuality will be eliminated as a defining charac-teristic of adolescents, a way of cutting and isolating, of separating and discriminating—is within reach. Yet there's a gap between what is being achieved in the real world of contemporary teenagers and what is acknowledged by researchers and scholars, mental and physi-cal health professionals, educators, religious leaders, policy makers, service providers, and parents.

I cannot, therefore, rejoice unreservedly, feeling satisfied or vindi-cated, as I write about these changes. Professionals are not my only audience. I write also for young people who are influenced by these professionals. I write for "pregay" young people, in the hope that they will never have to "act gay" or mold themselves into a stereotype or feel that their personal integrity must be sacrificed. If they can be convinced to relegate the idea of gayness to the dustbin, its previous existence forgotten except by those who will ask "What was *that* all about?", then the lives of millions of teenagers will be enhanced.

This book puts forth my argument and the supportive evidence, presenting a capsule summary of what we know and don't know about the lives of gay young people, from their first awareness of feel-ing different, to their first same-sex attractions and sexual experi-ences, to the point where they decide whether to put a label on their sexuality. Some of this evidence may be true despite the fact that our perspective is severely limited by the way in which this informa-tion has been obtained. Research has focused almost exclusively on the lives of those we might say are most gay—those most likely to feel compelled, for whatever personal or social reasons, to categorize their sexuality. Perhaps this has been unavoidable: those studying gay youth have naturally turned to those who are most visible and who are most willing to say, "Here, come interview me!" The result is that many other young people who are attracted to members of their own sex and who are not so flamboyant, who have been freed from the mandate to categorize themselves, have been invisible. No more.

My gratitude is greatest to the young people who have talked to me over the years, sharing their lives, trying their best to educate me. They've challenged my questions and my assumptions, they've forced me to better understand the limitations of my knowledge, and they've helped me realize the magic of their lives—how resilient they are, and yet how ordinary.

I am also grateful to my intellectual and professional home for the past thirty years—my university (Cornell University), my college (College of Human Ecology), and my department (Human Development)—for allowing me the freedom to pursue my scholarly interests. The gracious and patient staff of the Harvard University Press has been a dream to work with, especially Elizabeth Knoll, my senior editor, and Donna Bouvier, senior production editor. Finally, as he has for the past fifteen years, my life partner, Kenneth M. Cohen, continues to provide me with what I need to survive in good spirits.

THE NEW GAY TEENAGER

Why the *New* Gay Teenager?

The new gay teenager is in many respects the *non*–gay teenager. Perhaps she considers herself to be "postgay," or he says that he's "gayish." For these young people, being labeled as gay or even being gay matters little. They have same-sex desires and attractions but, unlike earlier generations, new gay teens have much less interest in naming these feelings or behaviors as gay.

I am not implying that young gay people have disappeared or that gayishness—behavior once thought characteristic of gay people—has taken over. Nor do I believe that homoerotic sex or love has been discarded. Rather, teenagers are increasingly redefining, reinterpreting, and renegotiating their sexuality such that possessing a gay, lesbian, or bisexual identity is practically meaningless. Their sexuality is not something that can be easily described, categorized, or understood apart from being part of their life in general. The notion of "gay" as a noteworthy or identifying characteristic is being abandoned; it has lost definition. As one self-described "pan-erotic" young man I interviewed put it, "'Gay' has been annexed and spandexed! It's been so bent out of shape that it don't exist no more."

Who are these revolutionaries? They are our students, our children, our younger sisters and brothers, and ourselves. Some we traditionally thought of as gay. Some we globally and conveniently referred to as "gay youth." We provided them with support groups, with Gay-Straight Alliances, and with therapy; we included them in our research. And this is how they thank us—by rejecting the very words we fought for? How can there be gay rights if there are no gay people?

Some of these new teenagers would admit to being "gayish" in their behavior or appearance. They might call themselves metrosexual boys or bi-anything girls. They might consider having sex with someone of their own sex, if they were asked or if the other person was really good looking or popular. They may even find themselves falling in love with someone of their own sex. They find same-sex encounters, alliances, and crushes appealing. They may be ordinary, boring teens, and yet they have so distorted "gay" to mean something more than sexuality and something less, something that has nothing to do with sexuality. For these new teens, "gay" carries too much baggage. One young woman told me in no uncertain terms, "If you want to know about me, don't ask about my sexual label like my mother did."

Perhaps we should ask, "Who's *not* gay?" These days it seems a lot of people want to get in on the act. After breaking up with Jennifer Lopez, actor Ben Affleck on *Saturday Night Live* displayed T-shirts for just about every possible romantic contingency, including one declaring "Ben-Gay"—"in the unlikely but wonderful hope that Matt Damon finally comes around." Singer Liz Phair boasts of "having gone lesbian" when she made out with a couple of girls in college. Women, she says, are "super foxy and turn me on." Acknowledging high ratings for his show, critical acclaim, and a high-profile magazine cover, Jon Stewart, host of *The Daily Show*, joked, "Are you saying we're the new gay?"[1] Even as "gay" loses its meaning, gayness is everywhere.

As we attempt to understand young people with same-sex attractions, this book provides a review and an interpretation of what we currently know. I first present evidence that has led me to believe that now is an appropriate time to rethink the nature and significance of same-sex sexuality among contemporary young people. In Chapter 2, I address the most perplexing question that confronts scholars, educators, mental health professionals, and parents: Who is gay? Answers to this question have changed dramatically over time. As I describe in Chapter 3, gay adolescence as a field of study was invented in the 1970s and has been only modestly transformed in the following three decades. One big mistake has been the creation of universal, linear sexual identity models to represent the lives of "gay youth." These helpful household hints fail to capture the diversity and complexity of young lives and have led researchers and clinicians down wrong and destructive pathways. In Chapter 4, I critique these models and offer an alternative: a differential developmental trajectories perspective.

These discussions lay the framework for Chapters 5 through 8. In those chapters, I review the developmental histories of young people with same-sex attractions, from their first feelings of being different, to their recognition of their own sexual attractions, to their first sexual experiences, and to their interpretations of what these attractions and behaviors mean for their sense of self.

In Chapters 9 and 10, I return to several themes raised in this first chapter. I argue that same-sex-attracted young people are more diverse than they are similar and more resilient than suicidal. Many now resist or refuse to identify themselves as gay and are living ordinary adolescent lives. They're adapting quite well, thank you.

Who Are These New Gay Teenagers?

Questions that we researchers should have been asking ourselves became glaringly apparent to me during my interviews with a number of young women and men.[2] Consider the following remarks of a nineteen-year-old young woman in response to my simple question "How do you identify your sexuality?"

> This took me a while, like, in college. My second semester I had met people in this co-op and got involved in feminist activities like "Take Back the Night," so this kept me in contact with lesbians. With my short hair and clothes they just assumed I was gay. I didn't, but they did. I didn't care one way or the other.
>
> My best friend Bryan was developing a crush on me. Mom gave me this T-shirt that had a triangle and a rainbow and said "Ready or Not Here I Come," and I thought it meant I graduated from high school. I wore it, and Bryan e-mailed me next day if I was lesbian, and so I told him I was not straight. So, since I wondered about him and it seemed only polite, I asked about him, and a week later he said he was just attracted to good people but had never thought about whether that made him gay before then.
>
> So, who's gay? I don't know how you can tell. Am I? Is he? Aren't we all! Shouldn't we be—I mean, if we were really true to ourselves? . . . Who should care? My sister asked me after I had this mammoth crush on this girl if this was one experience only or am I really gay. [I] told her I was not controlling my emotions, but did this mean if I wasn't I was gay? I'm about as much gay as heterosexual, as the next person, or maybe I'm just a metrosexual man posing as female. We're very close, and I told her sex and romance was a big part of my life and [I] didn't want to restrict it.[3]

Is this young woman gay? Perhaps she is simply gayish. Her response raises several fundamental questions. Does one have to have particular emotions or engage in particular sex acts to be gay? When is one gay and when is one not gay? Does one have to know one is gay to be gay? Perhaps it's possible to be gay for a little while and then not be gay for a while—to be gay in some situations and not in others—to be serially gay / not gay / gay / not gay. What does being gay look like, anyway?

I can't answer these questions, and I doubt that most teens can either. More important, they don't want to. What's the point? When someone acts or when something is described as "so gay," what does it really mean? It's not obvious that the reference is always, or even usually, to anything remotely associated with same-sex sexuality. Besides, these young people think, if straight teens don't have to sexually identify, why should I?

In response to the probes of parents, friends, and researchers, some teens label their lives with a sexual term—or are pushed into doing so. Many resist the temptation, or they disrespect the notion. They think it's an adult thing, being gay, and they find it difficult to relate to. What exactly is the connection between their same-sex desires and what gay adults say they experienced when they were young? These new teens know they're not totally straight, and they don't want to be. Most are okay with it. Some are thrilled with their sexuality, but don't see why they must therefore label themselves as gay. Yes, they are sexually attracted to other girls or other boys, perhaps ever so slightly. Maybe their feelings are romantic but not sexual—or sexual but not romantic. That's not bad. It's natural. It gives them an edge, a certain mystery. It sets them off from their peers—and from us adults.

In some respects, these teenagers might relate better to their pre-labeled, pre-identified grandparents than they do with their gay-liberated parents or their gay-resigned older cousins. Women and men from previous generations might not have identified themselves as gay, but this does not mean that they led lives of self-deception, repression, and furtive, transient pleasure-seeking or that they and their culture were unaware of their attractions.[4]

On a staid Caribbean cruise, I met four women over the age of sixty during an afternoon "Friends of Dorothy" event. If you're not at least middle age, you probably have no idea that the "Dorothy" reference means "gay." These women knew. The four have been friends for years and have been with their respective partners for decades. All are vibrant, warm, witty, embracing, and sensitive retirees from educational and health-related professions. In our hours of conversation they never once referred to themselves as lesbians—and they gracefully ignored it when I did. They have never formally "come out" nor declared their sexuality to coworkers or family members; yet in their families they're known as Aunt Peg, Aunt Josephine, Aunt Elizabeth, and Aunt Jill. They're not accustomed to explaining their sexual and romantic entanglements to siblings, cousins, nieces, or nephews. They don't have sexual identities, and they don't want them. They're simply enjoying the fullness of their lives, writing, skiing, canning, and snorkeling. I understand the humanness more than the gayness of their lives. I imagine that contemporary teens who minimize the significance of sexuality in their identity might better relate to these four women than to baby-boomer parents.

If "gay" won't do, what's the alternative? How best to designate former gays, current gays, will-be gays, and want-to-be gays? Over the years, the options have been many:

Bent	Invert	Friends of Dorothy
Queer	Pervert	Gay
Bugger	Third sex	Lesbian
Dandy	Uranian	Bisexual
Fop	Homosexual	Sexual minority
Molly	Fag	LGB
Ganymede	Dyke	LGBT
Lavender aunt	Sissy	LGBTQ
Androphile	Tomboy	LGBTQ^2
Sodomite	Amazon	LGBTQ^{2}U

These words don't carry the same meaning for teens that they do for us, the precursors and recipients of gay liberation and lesbian avengers. Some young people have an idea of what *a* gay person or *a* lesbian is. To them, being gay or lesbian is primarily an identity commitment, as in: "I'm gay." "It's who I am." "It's what I label myself." Although some may appreciate the historic significance and sense of identity the word "gay" connotes, I believe few young people aspire to it. Rather, in creating their own identity, they often use multiple terms as a way to respect both their gender and their sexuality. Consider some recently coined options:[5]

Boidyke	Trisexual	Stem
Queerboi	Omnisexual	Trannyfag
Polygendered	Stud	Bi-dyke
Trannyboy	Down low	Multisexual
Transman		

A modern teen can also "act gay," although exactly what that means is anyone's guess. It may be used to signify a boy's acting like a girl or a girl's acting like a boy—but this isn't always, or even usually, the meaning of the phrase. Whether a teenager believes he or she has "gay characteristics" may determine whether he or she would respond affirmatively to the question "Are you gay?" The word "gay" can also have social and political implications. These are usually leftist—though the Log Cabin Republicans are notable exceptions.

Most young people see little need to link their sexuality to their personal identity, attitudes, values, politics, religion, or life philosophy. Some even see no need to link their sexuality to their sexual behavior and romantic lives. Most young same-sex-attracted young people engage in sexual activities with both sexes. When it comes to their love life, however, they tend to be somewhat more discriminating.

Alternative terms proposed to label same-sex sexuality are also problematic. Some activists have attempted to reclaim "queer" from its negative connotations. However, "queer" describes sexuality less than it suggests one's philosophical, political agenda or lifestyle. After all, heterosexuals can be queer. After interviewing a number of young people over the years, Lisa Diamond concluded that "queer" as an identity never caught on. It flashed in the 1990s and then burned out.

"Sexual minority" is perhaps a suitably inclusive term, if narrowly defined. Unfortunately, it can also be easily misunderstood. Is someone who prefers sexual relations with a nonhuman animal a member of a sexual minority? Can a virgin be considered part of a sexual minority? The term also makes a questionable assumption: that non–sexual minorities—presumably, people who are exclusively heterosexual—are a majority. Finally, "sexual minority" is not a term that rolls easily off the lips.

Initials, as in "LGB" (or is it LBG? and why not GLB, GBL, BGL, or BLG?), can be handy. But who can agree on which initials should be included, or in what order? Also, initialized identities lack pizzazz. It's difficult to become emotionally attached to an L, a G, a B, a T, or a question mark.

Another option is simply to describe what is being referenced and not use a label. If I'm interested in the sexual behavior of an adolescent, for example, I would distinguish same-sex from opposite-sex behavior and anal from vaginal intercourse. If I want to know about the person's identity, I would say, "Pick [or create] a label." If sexual orientation is the critical component of my inquiry, I would determine the direction of the person's erotic fantasies and romantic attractions. Such assessments allow me to describe an individual who has varying degrees of same-sex behavior, same-sex identification, and same-sex attraction. I realize, however, that each of these sexual domains has its own share of problems. For example, What is sex? Is "unlabeled" an identity? What about those who feel no attractions? I explore these questions in the chapters that follow.

Descriptive terms, such as "same-sex attracted" and "homoerotic," name particular aspects of sexuality. They encourage discussion of a spectrum of sexualities rather than specific sexual categories. I also prefer them because of their neutrality and serviceability, their simplicity and naiveté. An individual can be homoerotic in some sexual domains and not in others. Similarly, one can be little or greatly same-sex attracted, in varying degrees and in varying ways. Using descriptive terms for the behavior includes gay, lesbian, and bisexual young people as well as those who refuse or resist labels for sexual identity. It also includes a person's having one or many same-sex encounters. So, too, virgins who would like to have sexual and/or romantic relations with others can be included. A teen with same-sex attractions can feel separate from straight and gay adult-centered worlds, or feel part of them. Describing same-sex behavior, feelings, and attitudes carries neither positive nor negative qualities, although some teenagers would disagree with this assertion, given the negative views of homosexuality in their own world.

But these are topics explored more fully in later chapters. First, let me introduce Scott and Abie, two young adults who typify their generation's diversity.

SCOTT

Scott came out of his life-long closet less than a year before I interviewed him.[6] The first person Scott told was Mike, his best friend, who provided him with a spiritual and a physical relationship. Next was the social worker assigned to Scott after he was admitted to his hospital's psychiatric unit. He had consumed a nonlethal dose of sleeping pills after Mike informed Scott that their sexual and emotional relationship had to stop because "God wants us to be pure."

Scott was eighteen years old when we talked, a rail-thin, blond young man of Scottish-German ancestry who lived in rural Vermont with his born-again parents and a drug-abusing younger brother. With his academic and creative accomplishments, Scott was the family's imminent hope for working-class escape. Aware since age seven of his intense physical and emotional attraction to boys, Scott had his first sexual relationship at the age of ten with Jim, whom Scott described as "my dorky friend who came out in junior high." Because of Jim's "swishy ways," their friendship raised suspicions about Scott's sexuality to his parents. Jim's "eighth-grade eight shades of lipstick" were difficult to ignore. Scott's parents eventually broke up their friendship because "Jim is too sick in the head."

By age twelve, Scott felt the full force of his same-sex erotic attractions. But he dared tell no one. Although he knew he had "homosexual tendencies" and wet dreams, he couldn't be gay! Maybe his attractions were gay, but he wasn't. His friend Mike told him that their all-night cuddling was an expression of their "Brotherhood in Jesus Christ" and that, according to the Bible, semen was to be expelled not through sex with girls (evil outside marriage) or masturbation (always evil), but with another Christian boy.

After the suicide attempt and several sessions with his social worker, Scott admitted that he was "probably bisexual" but that he would marry and have children. One year later, Scott said that he was "probably 100 percent gay" and was testing the waters of male-male sex and romance with contacts made through a college support group and the local gay bar.

ABIE

A college sophomore majoring in public policy, Abie recently "hooked up" with several boys. The sex was "reasonable," she tells me during the interview, but not particularly fulfilling. What to do with the guilt she feels the next day? She uses boys for her own "selfish hormonal purposes." But, then again, "They're all assholes." She doubts that the emotional caring she longs for can be found with boys.

A month ago, Abie felt gentle and yet fiery passion when she "went to Pennsylvania"—that is, got involved with Penny. The two spent hours together, telling each other their life stories and predicting their future. When not in daily face-to-face contact, they're in cell-phone contact. "This isn't sexual," Abie says somewhat defensively. Since eighth grade Penny has had sexual and romantic relationships with both girls and boys. But she isn't lesbian or bisexual, Abie tells me, because Penny told her, "Love depends on the person." Besides, Abie explains, "We're just best friends."

Abie assumes she's straight but confesses that she has never actually defined her sexuality. She has not "come out" to anyone because there's nothing to explain. But Abie became very confused when, after a party, she and Penny "messed around" when Penny slept over. The next morning Abie needed reassurance from Penny that their physicality meant nothing and would not impinge on their friendship. Once Penny reassured her, and with their emotional intimacy and trust intact, Abie feels no need to question her sexual status.

During the interview, I ask Abie about her sexual identity: "Is it the romantic, emotional aspect you want and not the sexual part? Does any of this have any relevance for your sexual identity?"

"So, you're saying I'm gay?" she responds. "I don't feel gay."

"How do you now identify?"

"I don't. What's the need?"

"But if you had to choose, what would you say?"

Exasperated, she says, "I don't. I don't have to choose. Why do you need to know?"

"I don't."

"All right, how about 'unlabeled'?"

In closing, Abie tells me in an ironic, even amused, but clearly not anxious, tone, "If only Penny had a penis, I'd be set!"[7]

SCOTT AND ABIE

Scott and his Mike conformed to a traditional mind-set. Abie and her Penny are part of the revolution. These four young adults represent the poles of contemporary youthful same-sex desire. Their elders, both gay and straight, may find Scott and Mike easier to understand. These two young men came of age in the early 1990s, when "gay youth" began its historic ascendancy and made its appeal for sympathy and attention. During this decade the caricature of the gay adolescent as a drug-abusing, hustling, sexually promiscuous, suicidal, runaway reject reached its zenith. Scott fits this image. His predicament was the seemingly inevitable consequence of being a vulnerable adolescent in a sexually prejudiced America. Perhaps the characterization was true in the early 1990s—or perhaps even then the image was overdrawn.

Abie and Penny, by contrast, are young women of the twenty-first century, a time when change and inconsistency are the norms. They and their friends, some of whom regularly hook up with guys, watch TV shows like *Queer as Folk, Totally Gay, Queer Eye for the Straight Guy, The L-Word*, and reruns of *Buffy the Vampire Slayer*. They watch these shows not for the political message or social commentary, but for the humor, the fashion tips, and the music. Abie and Penny are the new face of what may be called the disappearing gay adolescent. Maybe they're gayish. Maybe they're the new gay adolescent.

Scott and Mike and their gay male friends, now in their mid-thirties, do not understand Abie and Penny. They are of (at least) two minds. Scott is alarmed by the matter-of-fact appearance of gay characters in mainstream television and appalled by the political poverty of it all. To normalize gay is to castrate gay, in Scott's opinion. Will of *Will and Grace*, for example, is not gay because he's not having sufficient sex. Mike is embarrassed by the stereotypes of *Will and Grace*, but he's afraid that flaming Jack might be *too* gay and alienate straights by presenting the "wrong image." He is deeply mortified by the nudity and overt gay sex in *Queer as Folk*, hates the term "queer," and blushes over the gay makeovers of the Fab Five on *Queer Eye*.

This cultural divide is not between gays and straights or even among the various stripes of gay people. Neither is it between lesbians and gay men, blacks and whites, rich and poor, or urban and rural. Rather, as anthropologist Margaret Mead argued nearly forty years ago on the eve of the Stonewall Riots that marked the beginning of gay liberation, it is between generations.[8] In Mead's prefigurative culture, peers replace parents as models of attitudes and behavior. In such a culture, the present is not prepared by the past. It is a time in which young people are the real pioneers in a world community, immigrants in a new order of rapid cultural evolution. According to Mead, young people "feel that there must be a better way and that they must find it." Principles of fairness, equality, and libertarianism replace tradition, sacred texts, and cultural teachings.

A recent example illustrates the generation gap. All age categories in the United States oppose same-sex marriage save one. High school and college students shrug off the pollster's question, asking, "What's the big deal?" If their age group could and did vote, we would have a greater number of same-sex marriages, adoptions by same-sex couples, gay people serving openly in the military, sex-neutral civil rights, and openly gay presidents. To paraphrase the earlier question: "What's the difference?"[9] One commentator suggested, "What we may be witnessing are the beginnings of a cultural paradigm shift." Older generations are being replaced by younger generations who have more nontraditional or secular attitudes toward marriage.[10]

The fact that previous notions of "gay" are disappearing raises my hopes. Perhaps the end of gay adolescents as we think of them today is in sight. The possibility that contemporary teenagers are designing something new and better is the impetus for this book, though it concentrates on providing a history of what we thought we knew about "gay youth." The opportunity to know and accept the spectrum of same-sex-attracted, -behaving, and -loving teens has never been greater.

Cultural Makeover

In this new century, same-sex-attracted teenagers are leading lives that are nearly incomprehensible to earlier generations of gay youth.

To understand what it's like being young with same-sex attractions now often means discarding our previous ideas about what it means to be gay. We can't know about these adolescents' lives by looking at the experiences of their older gay brothers and lesbian sisters. Indeed, researchers studying gay adolescents should acknowledge the fragility of their findings because aspects of their data are old news by the time they are published. For example, the age at which developmental milestones are reached become younger with each generation sampled. At best, the lives of previous cohorts are merely guideposts, not authoritative texts about the life-course trajectories of today's young people.

The rapidity of the cultural makeover since the birth of the modern gay era has been nothing short of astonishing. Although Ellen DeGeneres's 1997 coming out on national television may be seen as a generational marker of progress, by now it seems ancient. It has been eclipsed by what columnist Maureen Dowd characterized in the *New York Times* as 2003's "Giddy Summer of Gays." She expressed sympathy for President George W. Bush, "stranded in his 1950's world of hypermasculinity as his country goes gay and *metrosexual* (straight men with femme tastes)."[11] Yes, regressive social beliefs, institutions, and Supreme Court justices remain (though teens are probably less concerned with these forces than gay adults believe they ought to be). And yes, young people are not sufficiently appreciative of what previous generations of gay people have done for them.

The younger generation is reasonably optimistic because a sea change has occurred, as reflected in polling data. The number of those who believe that sex between same-sex adults is "almost always wrong" has dropped nearly 20 points in the past decade.[12] The percentage of U.S. women who report having sex with other women has increased fifteen-fold since 1988. At least partly because of more positive images of gay people in the media and recent legal victories (most notably in the Supreme Court), it is now "easier for people to recognize their same-gender sexual interest and to act on it."[13]

Other evidence of this change in attitudes is to be found in popular culture. The September–October 2003 issue of *Bride's* magazine offered its first feature on same-sex weddings as Canadians in British Columbia, Quebec, Yukon, Manitoba, and Ontario plan their legal same-sex marriages. Madonna and Britney Spears lock lips at the MTV Music Video Awards, without loss of prestige or record sales.[14] Gay turns in movie roles do not diminish the careers of actors Jennifer Lopez, Meryl Streep, Russell Crowe, and Matt Damon. Television's *Will and Grace* and *Queer Eye for the Straight Guy* attract large audiences. Modern gay films seldom "plea for the straight world's tolerance of gay and lesbian sexuality" but routinely assume "a place where total acceptance is already a given."[15] The contrast between contemporary cinema and the seminal gay film of my young adult years, *Boys in the Band,* with its stereotypes, pleas for pity, and harrowing forecasts, is striking.

In business, nine of the top ten Fortune 500 companies have policies prohibiting discrimination based on sexual orientation. Even Wal-Mart, the nation's largest private employer and one of the most conservative mainstream corporations, includes sexual orientation in its antidiscrimination policy. Justifying their new policy, a spokesman for the company said, "We're clearly stating our acceptance for all of our associates."[16] The number of large U.S. companies that has received perfect scores for their fair treatment of gay employees, according to the Human Rights Campaign, doubled during 2003.[17] Civic leaders in many cities—not just gay meccas, but places such as Bloomington, Pensacola, and Philadelphia—roll out the "rainbow carpet" to woo gay tourists and their dollars. If not actively embracing gay people, these cities are at least learning to tolerate them.[18]

The most important legal case regarding gay rights was decided in 2003, when the U.S. Supreme Court, in Lawrence v. Texas, struck down sodomy laws. Justice Anthony Kennedy wrote that gay men "are entitled to respect for their private lives" and that "the state cannot demean their existence or control their destiny by making their private sexual conduct a crime."[19] City officials, mayors, governors, and other keepers of the law throughout the United States have openly challenged laws forbidding same-sex marriage.

Recognition of gay families has led to the integration of neighborhoods throughout the country, often silently, even imperceptibly. The gay-gentrified Boystown area of Chicago, the nation's first city-designated gay business district, has much in common with traditionally Republican Wheaton, Illinois.[20] Although both gay and straight adults sometimes struggle to find comfort zones of mutual respect and cooperation, they do exist. Conflict is considerably lower than anyone could have imagined in earlier decades. And assimilation in turn enhances acceptance through personal contact and the shattering of stereotypes. Straight people realize that gay adults also have children, give to charity, worry about trash pick-up, attend religious services, and maintain nice lawns.

Religious institutions have also been profoundly affected by cultural changes in attitudes toward gay people. Few other issues besides the inclusion of gay people in the life of the church or synagogue have so deeply divided American religious institutions. The Episcopal Church ordained its first openly gay bishop, Gene Robinson of New Hampshire, as the Presiding Bishop noted that Scripture does *not* condemn the love, forgiveness, and grace of committed same-sex relationships. The confirmation of Bishop Robinson merely acknowledged "what is already a reality in the life of the church and the larger society of which we are a part."[21] The ordination of openly gay individuals is a topic commonly discussed these days among mainstream Judeo-Christian denominations.

These examples illustrate striking progress in the treatment of homoeroticism. As the dominant culture assimilates what remains of gay culture, same-sex attracted adults routinely absorb and blend into the heterosexual mainstream. This happens, social critic Michael Bronski notes, because heterosexuality today is less often defined by inevitable procreation and marriage and because gay sex and gay people are less often viewed as immoral or unnatural. As a result, points of contact are less trepid.[22] Many of the supposed ill effects of being gay are leftovers from previous generations, who were affected by the cultural and interpersonal stigma and prejudice of the 1950s, 1960s, and 1970s.[23]

Today, no particular "gay agenda" exists, and sameness with the mainstream trumps differentness. Perhaps this has always been true. In some circles, "gay" has become merely another marketing niche to exploit. The gay image is less edgy, less different, more integrated; as Massachusetts Representative Barney Frank unapologetically admits, "I've been fighting all my life for the right to be boring." Young people would agree with him. To be treated like everyone else is the new revolution.[24] Dare I propose that the ultimate goal is to recognize the ordinariness of having same-sex attractions?

Whether this melding of previously separate gay and straight cultures is inevitable, unavoidable, or even desirable is a controversial topic. It is not just cultural conservatives who fear the inevitable. Some gay activists also long for the days when they could live their lives apart from mainstream culture. This debate among gay people about the desirability of gay-straight integration has recently flared up in the controversy over extending marriage rights to same-sex couples. Gay people both detest and long for marriage. Each side can recite philosophical and political rationales for their position. Those most politically involved in the battle for gay rights frequently regret the homogenization that aping straight culture is doing to gay people. Gay culture, they say, is better because it is less sexist, less classist, and less racist than heterosexual culture. Getting married is selling out to heterosexuality. Others want marriage because it represents true equality. Civil unions and domestic partnerships are not the same, they argue. Such compromises ghettoize gay people and make them feel like second-class citizens.

In describing this cultural clash, an article in the *New York Times* framed the debate on same-sex marriage in the following manner:

Many gays express the fear that it will undermine their notions of who they are. They say they want to maintain the unique aspects of their culture and their place at the edge of social change. It is a debate that pits those who celebrate a separate and flamboyant way of life as part of a counterculture against those who long for acceptance into the mainstream.[25]

By acknowledging this dispute, both sides seem to agree on one point: that a distinctly gay perspective exists.

Among teens, however, even this assumption is suspect. Such questions as "What is our nature?" "What is in our best interest?" and "What is the gay view?" are deliberated by adults, seldom by adolescents. The new gay teenagers rarely consider such questions. Their world is permeated as never before by tolerance, if not by outright acceptance. For many, same-sex desires are natural. Such young people can, but often choose not to, understand any other alternative. Many of their heterosexual peers agree with them.

What has fueled this dramatic generational shift? Probably the media, although little is known about how the media actually affect adolescent sexual attitudes and behavior. Conservatives accuse the media of depicting permissible and diverse (read: bad) sexual realities and expectations that normalize homoeroticism.[26] In reality, the media's rather paradoxical role has been both to silence and to publicize youthful same-sex desires. Even as an avalanche of scientific reports about suicidal, depressed, HIV-risky, substance-abusing gay teens became ubiquitous, MTV's *Real World, Road Rules,* and *True Life* introduced us to healthy, resilient, attractive gay teens who are shown to have the same basic needs as all adolescents. The cast members who are homophobic, refusing to tolerate their same-sex-attracted peers, are the deviant ones. The success of the entertainment industry in presenting and hence normalizing same-sex desire has had an incalculable impact on the ability of adolescents to understand their own emerging sexual attractions. Perhaps this alone has been sufficient to counter the doom-and-gloom perspective favored by academicians and health professionals.

Another change agent is in the public school system. In 1984, biology teacher Virginia Uribe developed Project 10, an in-school program to sensitize and educate staff on the presence and needs of gay students.[27] Similar efforts followed, first in Massachusetts schools in 1989; these evolved into today's Gay-Straight Alliances (GSAs), providing a safe space in nearly 2,000 schools nationwide for sexually questioning, gay-identified, gay-allied, and same-sex-attracted students. Supported and publicized by the Gay, Lesbian, and Straight Education Network (GLSEN), GSAs aim to provide counseling and support through the creation of "safe spaces" for gay students who are harassed or feel threatened; raise awareness among school personnel about gay issues and the destructive forces of homophobia; and increase the visibility and education among students and staff about gay issues in secondary and middle schools. Each GSA assumes its own unique structure, agenda, and membership constellation based on community standards and needs. Many include a large number of straight-identified (but not necessarily totally straight) allies.[28]

Within the past five years, GSAs have proliferated at an accelerating pace. Not uncommonly, early adolescents, aware of their nonheterosexuality, join as soon as they enter high school, and their friends and allies rally to support them. The popularity of GSAs has aroused controversy. Some conservatives argue that GSAs encourage homosexuality and provide a meeting place for their sexual activities. Liberals fear that GSAs serve to identify those who are gay, which places them at increased risk of becoming targets of antigay violence. Young people, however, appear far more nonchalant; they are untroubled by these adult anxieties. After all, gay-identified adolescents report that only 5 percent of the students in their school respond negatively to their sexuality; 95 percent are either positive or neutral. Whether GSAs are to some degree responsible for this level of acceptance is likely, but not proven.[29] In fact, though only a very small minority of same-sex-attracted teens choose to attend a GSA meeting, the visibility this organization gives nonheterosexuality is priceless.

These contemporary transformations have given gay people increased visibility and acceptance, but they have had unexpected ramifications. For example, with the increased cultural attention given to homosexuality, straight-identified teens, especially boys, seem to be more self-conscious when changing their clothing in public places. They are more apt to wrap towels around themselves as they head for the shower after gym. They fear that others of their sex might view their body with sexual lust. Previously, heterosexual boys had assumed the erotic privilege of viewership to be solely theirs. They could gawk, gape, and ogle girls' breasts and become aroused, but it never occurred to them that boys might erotically gawk, gape, and ogle at (read: evaluate) their "package." And girls have always known that boys were staring at their breasts lasciviously, but not that other girls might do the same.

I also suspect that straight-identified teens are becoming less likely to report and perhaps to engage in same-sex behavior. Homosexuality is everywhere nowadays! Aware of this, teens may no longer feel that sex with a best buddy is meaningless, that it is not a sign of homosexuality. When I was thirteen, it was considerably easier to excuse such behavior as just sexual experimentation springing from a sense of curiosity, fun, or an overindulgence in alcohol. For contemporary teens, same-sex behavior may mean much more.

These changes have had more positive results as well, symbolized, perhaps, by the straight young man who is happy to be made over by the Fab Five. The new, softer, gentler, emotionally sensitive young male is more likely to admit that he is "a little bit" attracted to particular men or that it's okay to act "gayish." We'll know that change has truly taken hold when thirteen-year-old boys who are best buddies, spend all their time together, draw hearts with their names in them, and profess their friendship and love forever are deemed as normal as thirteen-year-old girls who do the same.[30]

The Future

As I argue in the last two chapters of the book, I believe that the gay adolescent will eventually disappear. Teens who have same-gendered sex and desires won't vanish. But they will not need to identify as gay. They may not even need to have a predominantly or even significantly same-sex orientation. Disconnects between behavior, identity, and sexual orientation already coexist easily for many teens. Young women have been afforded this freedom for centuries, without being ostracized as gay.[31] They have been assisted by a philosophy (feminism) and a lifestyle (sex to express emotional attachment) that separate behavior, identity, and sexual orientation. Men loving men is not perceived the same way as women loving women—although maybe it should be.

Historian and political activist John D'Emilio has made many of these points on a larger sociopolitical platform.[32] He attacks the identity politics of the gay community, in part because it results in an us-versus-them mentality. Focusing on uniqueness blinds gay people to the possibility of building coalitions with subsets of heterosexuals, such as women, people of color, and immigrants. The dramatic cultural revolution of recent years, D'Emilio notes, affects the lives of people both gay and straight. Yet this fact seems to have gone unnoticed by gay activists who seem intent on imposing their radical politics on all nonheterosexuals. As a result, gay adults have stopped listening to their gay children, to the new generation. Unsparing in his criticism of those who glorify gayness as a means of identification, D'Emilio favors not gay marginality but the incorporation of the social changes won by gay people into existing institutions and mainstream politics. D'Emilio, however, appears to be unaware that, at least on a personal level, young people have already made these transformations and are living the dream of their gay elders.

Thus, what we should be heralding is the integration and normalization of homoeroticism, resulting in the near disappearance of the gay adolescent and the emergence of sexually diverse young people. We must move away from the pathos of gay teens to a recognition of their pride and resiliency and, eventually, of the *ordinariness* of same-sex-attracted individuals. The "new gay teenager" reinterprets gayness to signal the end of being gay. It is my hope that in the future, all books on the subject of "gay youth" will be history books. Young people who are resisting and refusing a specifically gay identity are making this hope a reality.

2

Who's Gay?

You probably believe you'd know a gay person if you saw one. Chances are, you're basing your judgment on particular characteristics that you've learn to associate with being gay. Maybe the person you spotted is gay. But what about all those you'd miss—those who don't fit your image? And what about the ones who fit your image but aren't gay? Who really is gay, anyway?

Researchers, educators, and mental health professionals "invented" gay adolescence in the 1970s and then watched it flourish in the 1990s. Gay adolescence came to be what we researchers wanted it to be—what we were. It looked remarkably like the adolescence of the researchers who were themselves gay—tough, difficult, painful, secretive, mysterious. Indeed, many of the early gay youth subjects were found in difficult circumstances—in support groups, psychiatric offices, and homeless shelters, perhaps on the streets. Those in attendance at gay youth support groups, for example, likely identified themselves as gay from an early age, came out to many, had an active sexual life, abused substances, and reported a high rate of personal and emotional problems.[1] But is this representative of gay youth today?

It depends. When a fifteen-year-old girl says, "I'm gay," her words mean something specific to her. Even if that something is clear in her own mind, however, her meaning might not necessarily be the same as what another fifteen-year-old intends the words to mean. Researchers usually define their subject pool based on the response to a specific question about sexual identity:

How do you identify yourself? Check the appropriate box (check only one):
☐ heterosexual
☐ gay/lesbian
☐ bisexual
☐ don't know

A person might respond differently, however, if the question had been "Have you had sex with a person of your own sex?" A response to the first question would not necessarily perfectly correspond with a response to the second. Some girls, for example, have sexual contact with other girls yet don't identify as lesbian, and some lesbians are virgins or only have sex with boys.

In addition to identity and sex, other aspects of same-sex sexuality have been proposed as appropriate means of identifying who's gay. What about the boy who falls in love with his best friend? What if a girl fluctuates among several sexual identities? What about a teenager who isn't yet aware that he's a member of, or doesn't want to be a member of, or isn't willing to disclose his membership in what he sees as a stigmatized group? Attraction. Romantic feelings. Erotic feelings. Fantasies. Lifestyle. Dating. Affiliation. Which—or how many—of these features define one as gay? Indeed, defining just who is gay has been frequently debated, and these debates have resulted in little scholarly consensus.[2] After half a century of research, we still can't agree on how to count gay people.

1	2	3	4	5
Not at all heterosexual		Somewhat heterosexual		Very heterosexual

1	2	3	4	5
Not at all homosexual		Somewhat homosexual		Very homosexual

Figure 2.1   The Shively scale for physical/affectional preference (source: Shively & DeCecco, 1977)

The most frequently used (and misused) measure is the Kinsey scale, which is usually represented as a seven-point continuum, from exclusively heterosexual to exclusively homosexual. The original interviewers asked their subjects about "overt sexual experience" and "psychosexual reactions."[3] Since then, the Kinsey scale has been used in many ambiguous ways and for multiple purposes—to assess sexual orientation and sexual identity as well as sexual behavior.

Another well-known measure is the Shively scale (Figure 2.1). This measure relies solely on physical and affectional preference. A creative addition is Shively's notion that homosexuality and heterosexuality should each have its own continuum.[4]

Still other scales have been proposed. The Klein sexual orientation grid assesses seven dimensions: sexual attraction, sexual behavior, sexual fantasy, emotional preference, social preference, self-identification, and heterosexual or homosexual lifestyle.[5] Sell's scale measures sexual attraction, sexual contact, and sexual identity and includes a gauge of the intensity and frequency of sexual interests and behavior that an individual has toward both males and females.[6] Clinician Eli Coleman advocates nine dimensions, including current lifestyle, future conceptions of idealized sexuality, sex-role identity, and self-acceptance of one's sexual orientation identity.[7] Any assessment should appreciate the dynamism, fluidity, and diversity of sexual orientation, but rules on how best to decide the relative importance of each dimension are few.

Creators of these scales generally ignore whether adolescents attribute any importance to these dimensions. Had they considered this, they might have been surprised. A recent study with adolescent focus groups addressed the question "What is sexual orientation?"[8] Regardless of gender or sexual status, the respondents agreed that sexual orientation has two aspects:

Sexual attraction, which may be described as a sexual desire for being with a specific gender; or an intense internal, physiological desire for a particular gender or to a particular person or attribute (e.g., body part).

A desire to be in a primary romantic relationship, which may include being in love with someone, forming a long-term commitment, and/or wanting to have such experiences.

Equally noteworthy is what the teenagers asserted is *not* particularly important:

Who you have sex with.

Self-labeling (e.g., straight, gay, bisexual).

Sexual fantasies.

Ironically, the very domains deemed irrelevant by those being studied are the very qualities researchers are most likely to use as markers of sexual orientation.[9]

Important to a young person, but rarely measured, aside from the seldom used Sell scale, is the *intensity* of sexual feelings or behavior.

Is an adolescent who has occasional or weak same-sex desires, fantasies, or behavior as gay as an adolescent who is overwhelmed by the eroticism of these experiences? If not, then how intense do these feelings need to be before one crosses over from straight to gay? If an adolescent boy has sex with another boy once and enjoys it but not intensely, is he gay? What if he has sex with someone of his own gender three times and it's intense the second time but not the first or third?

Also significant, but rarely measured, is the relative balance among sexualities.[10] Can straight teens enjoy same-sex fantasies and sexual encounters without being gay? If an adolescent girl has attractions for other girls, does this mean that she has to relinquish her lust for boys, her sexual activity with boys, her straight identity in order to be gay? If so, that may be too much for a teenager to abandon. Perhaps she could think of herself as a little bit gay, maintaining a desire to be heterosexually married, but remaining a virgin. If she has too many seemingly contradictory feelings, is she screwed up? Must sexual identity trump all other aspects of sexuality?

The simple solution put forward by so many researchers—ask kids if they're gay or not—teenagers find laughable. They'll lie. They'll hedge. They won't understand. They won't know. Whether the many sexual domains overlap within an individual, are always temporally congruent, are dynamic or static, or remain consistent or inconsistent over the life course is so conceptually intricate a question that we generally give up and find the easiest way possible to assess sexuality: "Gay or straight?" But what do we do with the young man who responds "sometimes" to the question "Do you ever wonder whether you might be homosexual (gay, lesbian) or bisexual?" He's not straight or gay but "unsure."[11] What he is unsure about, and why, remain unknown.

Another solution researchers frequently use to define who's gay is simply to determine who attends gay organizations, marches in gay pride parades, reads gay magazines, has gay friends, or responds to a call for gay participants in a proposed study. The motivation, importance, or meaning of these activities for the individual is ignored. Also ignored is the fact that many nongay people do these things.

Researcher Theo Sandfort argues that what we know about gay people "depends heavily on the definition and operationalization of homosexuality adopted, and on the way the sample has been put together."[12] In other words, who researchers say is gay and who they chose to provide data determine the outcome.

Orientation, Behavior, Identity

In deciding what constitutes a gay adolescent, we are confronted with the practical, but critical, task of how to define the population. The three primary domains researchers use to define sexuality within a population are outlined in Table 2.1.

SEXUAL ORIENTATION

Sexual orientation is the preponderance of erotic feelings, thoughts, and fantasies one has for members of a particular sex, both sexes, or neither sex. If sexual orientation is caused by genetic factors, it is present from conception. If it is caused by biological or intrauterine environmental factors acting on the developing fetus, it begins prenatally. If it is caused by psychogenic or social factors, it dates from early childhood. We are uncertain which is true, although the evidence is strongest for the first two.[13]

Sexual orientation is generally considered to be immutable, stable over time, and resistant to conscious control. However much one might want it to be otherwise, neither prayer nor reparative therapy (nor bad research) can change sexual orientation toward one pole or another.[14] Rather, it is sexual identity and behavior, not orientation, that are most subject to conscious choice and thus fluid over time.

Sexual orientation influences, but is often independent of, sexual

Table 2.1 Domains of sexual definition

	Sexual orientation	Sexual behavior	Sexual identity
A matter of choice	No	Yes	Yes
Stable over time	Yes	Yes/no	Yes/no
Awareness	Yes/no	Yes	Yes
Uniquely adolescent	No	No	Yes/no
Categorical	No	Yes/no	Yes

conduct and sexual identity. Similar to those with an opposite-sex sexual orientation who do not identify as heterosexual, many with a same-sex orientation never identify as gay. The disconnect between sexual orientation and sexual conduct has been noted by developmental researchers. Psychologist Harry Stack Sullivan observed many years ago that some preadolescent chums routinely have sex with each other, and that this has little bearing on their future sexual status. Some psychologists are fond of believing that friends who occasionally have sex with each other are simply "experimenting" and are "really" heterosexual. Indeed, the eminent Eleanor Maccoby recently asserted that "a substantial number of people experiment with same-sex sexuality at some point in their lives, and a small minority settle into a lifelong pattern of homosexuality."[15] The failure to assume a gay lifestyle is not interpreted as the consequence of societal heterosexism. Rather, the young person's natural experimentation has ceased and his or her inherent heterosexuality is assumed.

It is true that the majority of young people who engage in gay sex are heterosexual—at least by self-definition—according to a study of Massachusetts and Minnesota public schools. In that study, just over half of all students reporting same-sex behavior identified themselves as heterosexual.[16] Further, many gay-identified college men with pre-adult same-sex behavior believed it "likely" that their partners were heterosexual.[17] Whether these straight teens with same-sex contact were totally heterosexual or whether they were lying, in denial, or misunderstood is a matter of conjecture. We don't know because we never bother to ask heterosexuals about the incidence or meaning of their same-sex behavior. What we do know is that one of the best predictors of an adult sexual orientation is childhood and adolescent sexual behavior. A gay-identified young person is more likely to report a same-sex experience than is a heterosexual young person.[18] The relationship, however, is far from absolute. Kenneth Cohen's dissertation data revealed that although over 90 percent of young heterosexual college men described consistent and exclusive attractions, behavior, and fantasies (including fantasies resulting in orgasm) for females, it was not 100 percent.[19]

In addition to its conflating sexual orientation with sexual behavior and identity, contemporary research is plagued with other problems. Most biological and social scientists assume a categorical sexual orientation, allowing them to contrast heterosexuals with homosexuals. The category of bisexual is often ignored altogether or folded into the gay group. Bisexuals are said to be confused, in a state of transition, not yet having decided just what they are. So researchers decide for them. They're really gay. Or, if they're "bisexual leaning gay," they're gay. If they're "leaning straight," they're straight.[20]

These scholarly resolutions to the problem of who's gay are seldom congruent with the way young people see it. Members of the younger generation doubt that their sexual orientation can be reduced to *either* homosexual *or* bisexual *or* heterosexual. In every study conducted to date that gives young people a choice, they describe various degrees of homoerotic *and* heteroerotic attractions. For them, being attracted to one sex or the other is not mutually exclusive, and being attracted to boys and to girls might well fall along separate continuums. One can be from zero to one hundred percent heterosexual *and* from zero to one hundred percent gay. If researchers' sexual orientation categories do not fit the reality of adolescents, which should change?

Another researcher's nightmare is young people who refuse to put themselves into the sexual orientation rubrics we've created for them. They don't answer the question. They mark "don't know" or "not sure." They write in words such as "none," "queer," or "all of the above." The numbers of respondents who do this can be quite staggering. In a study of Native American Indian students, nearly one quarter did not respond to the question regarding sexual attractions and sexual intentions. Researchers usually exclude such noncompliants from their studies[21]—though if there aren't enough gay participants for statistical analyses these difficult-to-classify youth (and bisexuals) may be counted as gay. After all, they didn't identify themselves as heterosexual. In one study, there were more "not sure" responses than gay, lesbian, or bisexual. Researchers thereupon created a "GLBN orientation"—the N for "not sure."[22]

SEXUAL BEHAVIOR

Sexual behavior may at first appear to be considerably more straightforward than orientation. Either you've had sex or you haven't. You should know if you have or haven't. Yet, on closer examination, problems emerge. First, adolescents are notoriously poor reporters of sex, and they are even more so when "sex" is not clearly defined. Over 10 percent of high school students (especially boys) who said they had penile-vaginal intercourse "reclaimed" their virginity when asked the same question one year later. Only one quarter reported the same date of first (undefined) sex one year later; most revised the date to a more recent one, making them older at the age they first had sex.[23]

Another problem is that when researchers ask about sex, they're usually thinking about the old standby, penile-vaginal intercourse. Even when not so explicitly stated, this is what they mean—and they assume that twelve- to eighteen-year-olds will know this. They don't. Thus, whether "sex" has taken place depends on who gets to decide what "sex" is—researchers or the ones having the sex. Certainly, the researchers' unquestioned formula "sex = intercourse" is being seriously questioned by teenagers of all sexual orientations.[24] This makes it difficult to elicit reliable answers to such questions as "Have you had sex?" and "How many sex partners have you had?" These definitions matter in terms of sexual health, HIV prevention, and whether one has positive religious standing.

Whether adolescents' understanding of whether they've had sex matches what researchers mean by having sex is especially pertinent for young women who feel that romance trumps genital considerations. Indeed, a number of feminist scholars question the gender neutrality of the "sex = intercourse" equation.[25] Intercourse, they argue, represents only one form of sex—and not necessarily even the most common, enjoyable, or significant form.

How sex-as-intercourse applies when both partners are of the same sex is particularly baffling. By this definition, many same-sex-attracted adolescents haven't had sex—especially with each other. They've had encounters they feel are sexual in nature, yet these don't count because they don't qualify as intercourse. Two girls cuddle, kiss, and fondle each other all night. Two boys have mutual oral contact with the other's penis. Have these two couples had or have they not had sex?

These young people (or researchers) may decide that this same-sex activity counts as sex, but exactly what is the same-sex counterpart to heterosexual intercourse? Is it what is most clearly analogous to heterosexual intercourse—penile-anal intercourse for males and digital-vaginal intercourse for females? A study of gay college students may be suggestive here. Young gay men were more likely than lesbians to consider deep kissing and touching breasts to count as sex, and to believe that orgasm was essential for sex to occur. Lesbians, by contrast, espoused broader definitions of sex. Over 95 percent of the women in the study believed that oral contact with genitals constituted sex. For college men, that kind of agreement was attained only at the level of penile-anal intercourse.[26] Similarly, heterosexual young people define sex more inclusively. A majority asserted that same-sex activity could result in a loss of virginity, especially if the participants identified as lesbian, gay, or bisexual.[27]

Clearly, for most adolescents sex cannot be defined as only one activity at the expense of others. It depends. In general, same-sex-attracted young people are more likely than their straight peers to deem a large variety of behaviors as "having sex." Perhaps this accounts for the common finding that gay people have lots of sex and lots of partners and that they start having all this sex at an earlier age than heterosexuals do.[28] The fact that gay respondents define "sex" more broadly is rarely considered when researchers interpret reports of sexual activity.

With no standards to "certify" particular activities as sex, two adolescents with identical sexual histories might respond in opposite ways when asked whether they've had sex. The best remedy is for researchers to describe specific behavior and keep the focus of their study in mind when developing language to be used in their surveys.[29] If they wish to study oral herpes, then ask about oral sexual behavior; if pregnancy, ask about penile-vaginal contact. Researchers might also give greater weight to qualitative interview data, allowing teenagers to tell researchers their own definitions of sex, rather than the other way around.[30]

If researchers were made aware of the multifaceted meanings that same-sex-attracted adolescents attach to their sexual behavior, perhaps studies could focus on questions that are truly the important ones:[31]

What must happen to have sex?
When does sex begin?
Is it behavioral? Emotional?
What is the progression of specific sexual behaviors?
What does it mean to have same-sex activity with another person?
Must sexual activity be consistent or inconsistent with one's perceived sexuality?

Must one enjoy the sexual activity?

How do trajectories of sexual meaning and experience progress over the life course?

In short, simple tabulations of isolated behaviors reveal relatively little about whether adolescents have or have not had sex.

In addition, the links between sexual behavior (however it is defined) and other domains of sexuality can not be understood independent of each other. The motivations that underlie sexual behavior play a part. Consider the adolescent boy who engages in mutual masturbation with a best friend, but doesn't consider it sex because, he says, "I'm not gay." According to him, no "real" homosexual behavior (i.e., anal intercourse) took place. He's not in love with his friend, so he can't be gay. Or let's say a young girl assumes she can be sexually active or lose her virginity only if she is vaginally penetrated by a boy, although she admits that she and her best girlfriend have "done everything under the sun that two girls can do." Same-sex behavior emanating from curiosity, drunkenness, and social pressure may mean nothing about one's sexual orientation—or it may mean everything. So, too, a young person can be either conscious or unconscious of his or her sexual orientation and engage in no sexual activity at all (however it may be defined). Virgins can have a variety of sexual orientations.

SEXUAL IDENTITY

Sexual identity is a socially recognized label that names sexual feeling, attraction, and behavior. It is symbolized by such statements as "I am gay" or "I am straight." Although the specific label chosen is a matter of personal taste, the options are limited by the pool of potential, socially constructed identities defined by the culture and time in which one lives. Such labels can change and take on new meanings over time. For example, we know today that a bisexual is not someone who has to have *equal* attraction for males and females or who has to have at any given time two lovers, one of each sex. Current controversies over identity labels include whether transexuality reflects a sexual or a gender identity, whether "sexual fluidity" and "unlabeled" are sexual identities, and whether idiosyncratic contemporary terms (e.g., "queerboi") are legitimate. Because personal identities of all sorts are negotiated during adolescence, sexual identity may be especially susceptible to transformation during this time.[32]

Despite the possibilities outlined above, researchers usually define sexual identity in a rather limited fashion, with few available options. Forced-choice options do not appeal to teenagers. What about young people who identify themselves using a sexual label not provided, such as two-spirit, polysexual, or ambisexual? What about those who span multiple identities, the bi-lesbian or the gay-curious heterosexual? And what about those who claim no sexual label at all, who wish to remain fluid in their sexuality?[33] In which identity category should they be placed? This is a growing problem to researchers, as adolescents, especially young women, invent new terms to reflect their reality.[34]

Trying to match personal and/or public sexual identities with the corresponding sexual orientation or sexual contact isn't easy. Adolescents who are anything other than heterosexual or who resist simplistic notions of sexuality are apt to embody many inconsistencies. Thus, not only are some same-sex-attracted individuals left out of predetermined identity categories, but also a given category may include a variety of sexual orientations and behaviors. Consider:

- A girl with a single sexual experience with a boy but none with girls says to herself and her best friends that she has bisexual feelings. She's not ready to publicly declare bisexuality as her sexual identity. Instead, she calls herself "lesbian" because she perceives greater support for lesbians than bisexual women among her friends.

- A teenage boy labels himself "straight" and doesn't know what to make of the crushes he develops on boys. He engages in sex with girls to maintain his public veneer of heterosexual identity while privately "messing around" with boys to satisfy his lustful desires.
- A college student with heterosexual attractions, a liberal political philosophy, and no sexual activities declares herself to be gay as an act of identification with an oppressed group.
- A gentle, sensitive young man who has always known that he has heterosexual attractions has sex with his male friends because he is "saving" himself for marriage. When asked, he declares himself to have no sexual identity.

Adolescents forego or delay sexual identification for a variety of reasons, both philosophical and practical. Perhaps the directionality of their sexuality is not yet sufficiently self-apparent or strong. Perhaps their suspected identity is not tolerable to them personally or socially acceptable. Indeed, today's teens self-label on average several years before high school graduation.[35] This implies that many do not label themselves until young adulthood, or never. Why they do not do so, or why they do not do so earlier, is anyone's guess (but we ought to find out).

Alternatively, a young person may be "out" to himself, for example, but has decided not to share this information with others—including researchers who may be asking intrusive questions in his high school classroom. Indeed, the mean age of disclosing one's gay identity to others is just before or after high school graduation.[36] Why not earlier? Perhaps a boy doesn't want others to see him as gay. Or he feels that he doesn't fit, nor does he want to fit, cultural definitions of gayness, such as the effeminate boy with purple, spiked hair. He may dislike the sexual and political associations of being gay, or may feel that the gay label is just too simplistic, too reductionistic to capture the full extent of his sexuality. He's more than gay. Gay boxes him in, constrains his options, and oversimplifies a complex aspect of himself. He might claim it for himself, but he doesn't want others to do so. Another boy might feel indifferent about being gay. It's just who he is. But he fears the potential life-altering repercussions if his gayness was to become public knowledge.

Thus, surveys and interviews miss many of those who will eventually identify as gay after adolescence and nearly all those who will never identify as gay but who nevertheless have a same-sex orientation and engage in gay sex.[37] These young people slip out of the reach of research studies, educational programs, support groups, and political rallies. One consequence of this is that what can be known about their lives, and thus about same-sex sexuality, is limited. These kinds of problems stand in the way of our learning even the most basic information—how many gay adolescents are there, anyway?

The Answer

How many? It depends. It depends on how we define the population—by attraction, behavior, or identity. Coming up with definitions is a rather precarious endeavor because, as we have seen, self-identified heterosexuals engage in same-sex behavior and have same-sex attractions, and most same-sex-oriented adolescents have a heterosexual sexual history and identity. A same-sex orientation is often unwanted and sometimes goes unrecognized during adolescence. This fact led a renowned group of sex researchers to conclude, "Estimating a single number for the prevalence of homosexuality is a futile exercise because it presupposes assumptions that are patently false: that homosexuality is a uniform attribute across individuals, that it is stable over time, and that it can be easily measured."[38] This has not, however, prevented us from attempting to do so.

An example of the problems inherent in counting gay people is nicely illustrated in a national, representative study of Dutch men.[39] Theo Sandfort reported the following based on various definitions of same-sex sexuality.

- 6 percent of respondents identified as gay or bisexual. Not surprisingly, all of the gay men in this group reported having same-sex physical attractions, sex, and love. Bisexuals were mixed, endorsing one or two but seldom all three of these components. One man who identified himself as bisexual reported feeling none of the three; on what basis he claimed to be bisexual is not clear.
- 7 percent of respondents reported being in love at least once with a man. All of these men reported having same-sex physical attractions, and nearly all had had sex with a man. Despite their homoerotic love, attractions, and sex, one in five of the 7 percent claimed to be heterosexual.
- 8 percent of respondents considered that they *might be* homosexual. All reported being physically attracted to men, and most had had sexual experiences with men. Over one third of this 8 percent said they were not gay.
- 13 percent of respondents said they had had sex with a man. One third of these men were not, however, physically attracted to men; about half identified as gay or bisexual or reported having been in love with a man.
- 14 percent of respondents reported feeling physical attractions toward men. Half of these noted that these feelings disappeared later in life; nearly all reported loving women. Two in five of this 14 percent had had sex with a man; under half reported never having been in love with a man.

What are we to make of this? Concluding that 6 percent of the population is gay or bisexual (the percentage so self-identifying) would be understating the total number of men who experienced at least some aspect of same-sex sexuality. Even the reported percentages might be conservative, given the stigma associated with homosexuality (even in the Netherlands). Studies of adults in the United Kingdom, France, and Australia found that almost 20 percent reported either same-sex behavior or same-sex attractions since age fifteen; but fewer than one third of these individuals identified as gay.[40]

Clearly, estimating the number of gay adolescents depends on what counts as gay.

IS IT ENGAGING IN SAME-SEX BEHAVIOR?

A truthful estimate of same-sex behavior is usually difficult to verify. The stigma attached to "homosexual sex" still reigns within adolescent culture. At the high end are the numbers Kinsey provided of adults reflecting on their sexual histories. Although 37 percent of men and 13 percent of women reported "at least some overt homosexual experience to the point of orgasm between adolescence and old age," only 10 percent of men and 4 percent of women were more or less exclusively homosexual for at least three years between the ages of sixteen and fifty-five.[41] A cross-cultural review of the evidence published a decade ago found half this rate. In addition, its author, Mickey Diamond, concluded that "most individuals, most of the time, and for most of their lives, have sex with only males or females, not both."[42] That is, sexual experimentation might last for several years, especially during adolescence or young adulthood when it's most acceptable and means the least; but it does not persist over a lifetime.

Studies of same-sex behavior among adolescents and young adults, however, have produced strikingly lower numbers than among adults. The U.S. rate is usually reported as being around 2 percent to 4 percent.[43] This proportion increases with age among teens—for example, from less than 1 percent among twelve-year-old boys to nearly 3 percent among eighteen-year-olds in one study.[44] Young people who have had prior heterosexual sex are also more likely to have same-sex contact; one study of Vermont students showed the percentages going from 1 percent among typical students to nearly 7 percent of those heterosexually experienced.[45]

Gender differences are nearly always found. More boys than girls report same-sex behavior. However, whereas half of boys quit sex with other males after adolescence, attributing their behavior to teenage curiosity or to sexual release, most girls with girl-girl sexual contact continue to pursue it into adulthood.[46] Hence women's adolescent sexual behavior is a better predictor of their adult same-sex sexuality than it is for young men. When heterosexually identified young women pursue sex with another female, they often do so in college rather than in high school, perhaps because girls have historically had fewer opportunities and social license to be sexually engaged during their adolescent years.[47]

The prevalence rate of same-sex behavior also varies in different cultural contexts. In studies of Greek and British young adults, about 3 percent reported same-sex activities.[48] An international survey of sixteen- to fifty-year-olds reported ranges from 6 percent of U.S. males to 11 percent of French males and from 2 percent of United Kingdom females to 4 percent of U.S. females. Very few adults in any country reported having exclusively same-sex experiences during the previous five years.[49] Thus, most of those who have sex with their own sex also have it with the other.

One undeniable, well-substantiated fact is that most individuals with same-sex contact during adolescence claim at the time to be heterosexual. This one fact poses enormous problems for sampling a representative population of "gay youth" if the basis for obtaining the sample is same-sex behavior. It's impossible to know how much of

Table 2.2   Sexual identity transitions of young women

	Defections	Adoptions
Lesbian	25%	19%
Bisexual	33%	23%
Unlabeled	33%	37%
Heterosexual	10%	21%

Source: Diamond, 2003b.

the reported same-sex behavior represents experimentation and how much emanates from the individual's sexual orientation.

IS IT IDENTIFYING AS GAY, LESBIAN, OR BISEXUAL?

Despite the substantial number of young people who have some component of a same-sex sexuality, less than 2 percent of high school students actually identify as lesbian, gay, or bisexual.[50] In addition, once an adolescent identifies as something other than straight, there's no guarantee he or she will keep that identity. Lisa Diamond found in her study of young women over an eight-year period that 60 percent changed their sexual identity at least once and nearly 50 percent gave up their lesbian or bisexual label at some point. Some reclaimed a lesbian or bisexual label, and some reclaimed a previous heterosexual label.[51] Bisexual and unlabeled young women were most likely to defect to another label. "Unlabeled" was the category most likely to be adopted (see Table 2.2).[52] It is not that these young women gave up their sexual attractions to women or considered their previous sexual identification to be simply a "phase." Typically, the relative intensity of same-sex compared to heterosexual attractions, coupled with a serious and satisfying relationship with a male, led the young women to identify as heterosexual. Even as they did so, they continued to acknowledge their ongoing potential for same-sex sexuality.

41

The usual interpretation of an inclination not to identify as gay is attributed to the stigma associated with a same-sex identity. Other possibilities are seldom considered, but will be in the last chapter of this book.

IS IT ACKNOWLEDGING A SAME-SEX ORIENTATION?

A national, representative sample of adults illustrates several well-documented truths. First, the proportion of individuals with same-sex attractions (8 percent) is considerably greater than the fraction who identifies as gay, lesbian, or bisexual (2 percent). Second, more have same-sex attractions than engage in same-sex activities (7 percent).[53]

Traditionally, among adolescents the numbers are lower, but the proportions remain constant. Although nearly 5 percent have same-sex sexual fantasies or have predominant sexual attractions for others of the same sex, just over 1 percent report same-sex behavior or a gay or lesbian sexual orientation identification.[54] Age can make a big difference in these numbers. In a study of public school students, the proportion of twelve-year-olds who reported a predominance of "homosexual attractions" was just over 2 percent and increased thereafter. The proportion doubled among the fifteen-year-olds and tripled to over 6 percent among eighteen-year-olds.[55]

FINALLY: THE ANSWER

A recent representative study of adolescents provides more helpful information about the frequency and consistency of various domains of same-sex sexuality across time.[56] Table 2.3 summarizes the proportion of adolescents who reported having same-sex romantic attractions, same-sex behavior, a same-sex orientation, and a gay or bisexual identity when they averaged 16 years, 17 years, and 22 years of age. (The latter two domains were only assessed at Time 3.)

Table 2.3 Domains over time

Sexual domain	Females			Males		
	Time 1	Time 2	Time 3	Time 1	Time 2	Time 3
Same-sex romantic attractions	5%	4%	13%	7%	5%	5%
Same-sex behavior	1%	1%	4%	1%	1%	3%
Sexual orientation:						
Mostly heterosexual			10%			3%
Bisexual			3%			1%
Mostly homosexual			1%			1%
Homosexual			0.5%			1%
Sexual identity:						
Gay			1%			2%
Bisexual			3%			1%

Source: Savin-Williams & Ream, in preparation–a.
Average age: time 1, 16 years; time 2, 17 years; time 3, 22 years.

Considering only the Time 3 data, how many gay young people there are depends on what one means by "gay." Among females, if "gay" is defined as same-sex behavior or a gay or bisexual identity, 4 percent of them are gay. However, if having some degree of same-sex attractions is the criterion, then there are over three times as many. Among males, if same-sex behavior or gay or bisexual identity is the defining factor, then gays number about 3 percent of the total. If the definition is same-sex attractions, then there are nearly twice as many.

These longitudinal data may be clouded by cohort factors. The picture may be changing. Traditionally, young people report about the same proportion of same-sex attractions and gay identification as adults, but somewhat less same-sex contact (after all, they've had fewer years of opportunity). The Time 3 data in Table 2.3 and the results of two recent studies indicate a new trend. Increasingly, a larger proportion of young people say they have same-sex attractions. In the Time 3 data, it was 6 percent (men) and 15 percent (women). Among college students in another study it was 10 percent (men) and 12 percent (women). Perhaps more indicative of the cohort trend, nearly 25 percent of women and 20 percent of men reported "any attraction" to the same sex.[57] Among high school students, 6 percent "know that I am homosexual or bisexual" and, more strikingly, 13 percent (twice as many girls as boys) sometimes or frequently wonder if they might be homosexual.[58]

Based on the evidence at hand, I conclude the following:

- Assuming that sexual orientation is determined prior to puberty, it is safe to conclude that at least 15 percent and maybe as high as 20 percent of all adolescents have some degree of a same-sex orientation.
- Less than half of these individuals are exclusively or near exclusively same-sex oriented.
- Teens with some degree of a same-sex orientation far outnumber the 3–4 percent who embrace a gay or bisexual identity or the 3 percent who report same-sex activities.

Discrepancies

Our understanding of how teenagers of any orientation experience sexuality is shockingly primitive. Neither do we know much about how their sexual domains connect in their lives. Sexual attractions are felt as physical arousal or erotic, romantic, spiritual, psychological, or emotional stirrings. Teens rarely mention their sexual behavior as the defining characteristic of their sexual selves. These disconnects are to be expected. Paula Rodríguez Rust reminds us that individuals can romantically fantasize about a girl while having sex with a boy, can flirt with a girl while secretly desiring her boyfriend, and can marry a man without giving up sex with a woman.[59]

I believe we must first assess each domain separately rather than implicitly treat one as a proxy for another. If your inclination remains the latter, consider the 1992 report of Minnesota students:[60]

- Just 1 percent had a same-sex sexual experience, but most of these individuals also had a heterosexual experience.
- Heterosexual sex was as likely to be reported by a gay- as a heterosexually identified individual.
- Of those with same-sex behavior, only 27 percent identified as gay.
- Overall, 1 percent identified as gay, although few of these individuals also reported same-sex behavior.
- Nearly 5 percent reported having primarily same-sex attractions; of these, only 5 percent identified as gay.
- The correlation between a gay sexual identity and a same-sex orientation was strikingly low—.1 for girls and .3 for boys.

If you remain unimpressed, unmoved by these statistics, and incredulous over the discrepancies, consider Figure 2.2. Designed by Lisa Diamond, it depicts the relationship between sexual attractions and sexual behavior among a group of young women she studied over a period of eight years.[61] The diagonal line represents perfect positioning between the two; the dots correspond to individuals in the study. There is a relationship between the two, but it is far from perfect.

Despite what we might wish, sexuality is rarely in perfect alignment during the teenage years and perhaps beyond. We shouldn't ignore these intricacies and inconsistencies of same-sex sexuality when they show up in our data or in the person standing in front of us. Yet what are we to do about them?

If the critical deterrents to understanding adolescent sexuality are the diverse meanings and connections attached to various sexual factors, then we need research that assesses these meanings and connections. How do young people of different sexual persuasions experi-

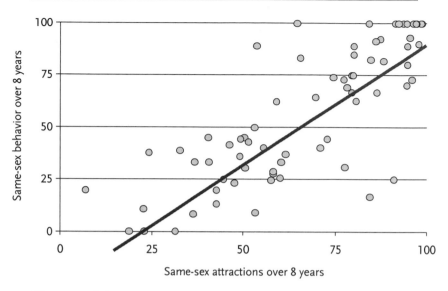

Figure 2.2 Relation between women's sexual attraction and sexual behavior

ence same-sex feelings, cognitions, and interactions? How do these experiences contrast with their heterosexual components? An innovative approach would be to recruit heterosexually oriented adolescents, especially those who report same-sex attractions and behavior, into the research.

Perhaps teens with greater levels of underlying same-sex orientation pursue same-sex activities more consistently and fervently and are more apt to choose them over opportunities for opposite-sex contact. This would be less true of bisexuals. For example, in the Vermont study of public schools, over half of the boys with a same-sex experience reported having not just one, but more than four different male partners. Slightly over half of the gay- or bisexually identified boys and three quarters of the lesbian- or bisexually identified girls reported engaging in heterosexual sex.[62] However, these encounters tend to be at a later age, with fewer partners, and for less "lustful" reasons than their same-sex encounters.[63] Among young women, the only significant predictor of a future same-sex identity was having more same-sex than opposite-sex attractions—which replicates the Vermont study if female attractions are substituted for male sexual behavior.[64]

Another useful effort would be to distinguish characteristics of adolescents who have a predominantly same-sex orientation and, of these adolescents, which ones engage in same-sex behavior or identify as a sexual minority. Perhaps some childhood indicators are better predictors of gay identification or same-sex behavior than others, or the more one has of these predictors the greater the likelihood of identifying as gay or engaging in same-sex behavior. Perhaps one's having particular characteristics reflects different sources of sexual orientation formation. The only childhood variable that has received even a semblance of attention has been the degree to which an individual possesses sex-atypical characteristics, either in sex-role motor behavior ("He walks like a girl"), personality ("She's so extroverted"), interests ("He plays with dolls"), or career ("She's an engineer"). Yet Lisa Diamond found that the typical childhood and adolescent factors that predict gayness among boys, such as an early age of first same-sex attractions, sex atypicality, and early age of first same-sex contact, were seldom in the histories of women with same-sex attractions.[65] Either the task of predicting female sexual orientation is more difficult or we have not yet unearthed the relevant childhood/ adolescent variables for young women. In either case, sensitivity to gender is clearly in order.

These matters are further complicated by cultural considerations. For example, paradoxical attitudes toward male-male sexual behavior are common in many Latino cultures, which may "permit" males to choose other males as sex partners provided that it is a private activity undertaken solely to satisfy sexual urges. Public expression of same-sex love or profession of a gay identity is much more controversial. Furthermore, a Latino man may pursue gay sex without threatening his heterosexual identity (to himself and others, including his sex partner) if he is the active agent in anal sex and the recipient of oral sex. He must maintain a highly masculine demeanor and express no tender feelings toward his partner (e.g., no kissing). Males who consent to being penetrated are often ridiculed as *jotos* (faggots).[66]

Ultimately, what is most needed, though it may be too difficult to achieve, is to gain in-depth qualitative information from teenagers about their sexual experiences and what they see as the meaning and significance of those experiences. The next best alternative would be to obtain such information from nonminor young adults who are just past the age of adolescence, away from home, on their own, but not too far removed from the relevant memories and experiences. The combination of greater maturity and exposure to diverse understandings about same-sex sexuality might make such respondents more willing to speak openly and honestly about their sexual feelings and experiences.

Most research on gay teens has, sadly, neglected the many others who have homoerotic feelings. As one researcher put it, this has led us to investigate "not homosexuality but self-identification as homosexual."[67] Thus, the vast majority of studies cited in this book are concerned with those who identify as gay, lesbian, or bisexual. This would not be a problem if these young people can truly represent those who do not so self-identify.

The present generation of adolescents gives us reason to doubt this assumption.

3

In the Beginning . . .
Was Gay Youth

The transition from there being no gay teenagers to lots of them virtually blindsided experts of adolescent development. It was a major coup for clinicians to invent gay adolescents, to establish an awareness and a sensitivity in their profession to such young people's existence. The evolving idea of the gay adolescent from its humble beginnings in the early 1970s has not been altogether inaccurate, despite the fact that experts, often with the best of intentions, have frequently presented these teenagers as hopelessly suffering and even suicidal. Unencumbered with this knowledge about how they are supposed to feel, act, and believe, millions of teens with same-sex attractions continue to live their daily life with as much happiness and angst as any other teenager.

Professionals' understanding of gay adolescence can be said to have evolved during four time periods:

1. *The 1970s and 1980s.* In the seventies and eighties, gay adolescence came to be recognized as a distinct category from "normal" adolescence, almost as if gay youth may constitute a separate species.

2. *The 1980s and 1990s.* In the eighties and nineties, gay adolescents are characterized with a "suffering suicidal" script; this is supposed to provide them with guidance as to what they should expect in their lives.

3. *The early 2000s.* Nowadays, the possibility that gay adolescents might include resilient, proud, and adaptive individuals is inching forward.

4. *The future.* We can hope that in the future, a specifically "gay" adolescence will not exist and that same-sex-attracted individuals are found to be rather quite ordinary, neither better nor worse off than other adolescents.

In the Beginning

Those on opposite sides of the biological-cultural divide regarding the invention of "the homosexual"[1] agree on one fact: that adolescents who are romantically and erotically attracted to others of their biological sex have always existed, in every recorded culture and in every historic time. Only recently, however, have young people incorporated these attractions into their sense of self, publicly announced their attractions to friends and relatives, and formed a personal identity based on their attractions. Gay adolescence is a modern invention.

The presence of preadult individuals with same-sex desires is well documented by social historians and anthropologists. Among girls, intense, erotic friendships are referenced in various cultures as "smashes," "mummy-baby friendships," and "passionate friendships."[2] Within this female world of love and ritual, girls acted out their unconsummated (we assume) emotional pinings. To us today, these pairings look a lot like love relationships. In their time and in their world, these same-sex romances were judged acceptable, in part because few could fathom that the girls might be having sex. What would they do? But even if the relationships lacked explicit sexual activity, they nevertheless contained passionate longings for spiritual, emotional, and physical contact. "We will always be together." "I'll share my life with you." "I want to kiss you all over." Emily Dickinson wrote such longings to her absent friend, Susie. She also wrote:

[I want you to] be my own again, and kiss me as you used to . . . [I] feel that now I must have you—that the expectation once more to see your face again, makes me feel hot and feverish, and my heart beats so fast.[3]

It's difficult to ignore the homoerotic character of this letter.

Boy-on-boy relationships, especially those explicitly genitally oriented, have been more easily understood, with a wink and a nod. English upper-class families, according to one source, often accepted youthful "homoerotic attachment as not only natural but desirable"—although such relationships were seldom publicly acknowledged. Some of these attachments evolved into lifelong sexual and romantic adult partnerships.[4] In Maya, parents not infrequently provided their son with a male companion, perhaps a slave boy, to "meet his needs."[5] In some Native American cultures, sex-atypical boys who were seen as having two spirits were held in high esteem because they were believed to have received the gift of both masculinity and femininity. Permitted to live as females, some took a male for a spouse.[6] And in Sambian culture, receiving the semen of a more mature male was considered a vital and virtually universal (mandatory) feature of becoming a man.[7] However, a certain number of Sambian men went beyond the usual custom by voluntarily offering their semen on a regular basis.

In the United States, following the publication of Alfred Kinsey's research in the 1940s and 1950s, it was difficult for anyone to assert that American adolescents were *not* having sex or *not* falling in love with others of their sex. Some adults admitted as much. Lord Baden-Powell, founder of the Boy Scouts, experienced same-sex feelings and behaviors during his formative years. According to him, these desires eventually disappeared. Baden-Powell wrote about the transitory nature of "impure" sexuality in the 1908 *Scouting for Boys* manual. He advised that these impurities could be eliminated with a plunge of one's "racial organ" into icy water.[8]

Another adult male in the public eye who was personally invested in minimizing the long-term consequences of adolescent homoerotic desire was the eminent psychologist and clinician Harry Stack Sullivan. He concluded that "mutual masturbation and other presumably homosexual activity" occurred not among those who eventually identified as "overt homosexuals" but among those (himself included) who eventually "married, with children, divorced, and what not, in the best tradition of American society."[9] Thus, sexual relations among childhood chums were of little concern precisely because they implied nothing about one's future sexuality.

Up to the early 1970s, the only face of gay adolescence was Lance Loud. The first star of reality television, Lance presented a real-life portrait of himself in the 1973 PBS show *An American Family*.[10] His silver-dyed hair, flamboyance, and pen-pal correspondence with Andy Warhol pretty much matched the stereotype the American public had of a "sexual invert." Lance was the unacceptable but expected gay adolescent.

The change in the visibility of homoeroticism between 1973 and today is nothing short of revolutionary. A young person nowadays cannot turn on the television without viewing gay characters, gay innuendos, gay themes, and gay advertisements. According a 2001 article in the magazine *American Demographics,* more parents than not say they talk with their children and adolescents about what it means to be gay. Three quarters of children in third to fifth grade are "very" or "kind of" comfortable talking to their parents about what it means to be gay. Among early adolescents, the proportion approaches 90 percent.[11]

What follows is a brief overview of four epochs of gay youth. In each period, the aspects of their lives deemed meritorious of investigation and the venues from which professionals have recruited study subjects have changed. How professionals chose to study gay youth has led to biases that still linger.

The 1970s and 1980s: Invention

Medical and mental-health clinicians began to note the existence and plight of gay teenagers in the early 1970s. Usually the subjects of their study were male adolescents in peril, prostitutes, runaways, and delinquents. These troubled, at-risk young people were the only gay teenagers who came to the notice of social service agencies and providers. No one particularly cared whether these adolescents were representative, or even typical, of other young people with same-sex attractions and behavior. In short, these troubled teens needed to be rescued, and by publicizing their destitute lives researchers hoped to put into place services that would best address the problems of these young people. The mere fact that these teenagers were located was itself notable.

The first empirical study of gay adolescence was published in 1972, in a medical journal. Sixty young men between the ages of sixteen and twenty-two, many of whom were Seattle hustlers, were the focus of the study.[12] Not surprisingly, given the study population, the respondents' number of sexual encounters with other males was very high, in some cases exceeding 3,000 partners. Most boys had gone to a gay bar at least once, were secretive about their sexuality, and felt rejected by society. Almost half had seen a psychiatrist or sought mental-health counseling. When asked what they saw as the greatest problem associated with homosexuality, the boys cited a lack of acceptance in the straight world and the repulsion they themselves felt toward other homosexuals. To the young men in the study, homosexuals are inherently distraught, desperate people because of what they are and how they must live. Morbid suicidality reflected the intense unhappiness of these young men. Emotional turmoil was a developmental necessity in establishing a gay image and lifestyle.

This one study stood as the sole empirical investigation into the lives of gay adolescents for fifteen years, until in 1987 medical clinician Gary Remafedi published two papers based on 29 boys between the ages of fifteen and nineteen.[13] Recruited through gay-oriented media and the local health department, Remafedi explored the stressors that placed the boys at high risk for physical and psychological problems. Indeed, most of Remafedi's subjects had experienced school truancy, poor grades, substance abuse, and emotional difficulties and had consulted a psychologist or psychiatrist. Nearly half at one point had had a sexually transmitted disease, had run away from home, or had committed a crime. Nearly a third had been hospitalized for mental-health issues and had attempted suicide. Most of the others believed they would try to kill themselves in the future. Despite this profile, Remafedi concluded that it was "unlikely" that his sample was skewed toward poorly adjusted adolescents. He believed that the "very experience of acquiring a homosexual or bisexual identity at an early age places the individual at risk for dysfunction."

At about the same time as such findings were being published, institutions devoted to gay teens were founded. Most notable was the Institute for the Protection of Lesbian and Gay Youth (IPLGY), formed in New York City in 1979 (now the Hetrick-Martin Institute and the affiliated Harvey Milk School). Soon, social services and community support groups were being established in other urban centers. These institutions aimed to address the critical physical, educational, therapeutic, and social needs of gay youth. They also provided for the first time a pool of potential research subjects.

One such study attempted to analyze the presenting problems of over 2,000 young people who telephoned seeking counseling and crisis intervention or who were walk-ins to the IPLGY service agency. Feeling cognitively, emotionally, and socially isolated, especially from family members, these young people faced violence, sexual abuse, and peer bullying. They had, the authors of the study found, "many symptoms of emotional disturbance [with] signs of clinical depression—pervasive loss of pleasure, feelings of sadness, change of appetite, sleep disturbance, slowing of thought, lowered self-esteem with increased self-criticism and self-blame and strongly expressed feelings of guilt and failure."[14] They felt alone in the world. They felt that no one else shared their problems and concerns.

Another team using the IPLGY clientele was led by Mary Jane Rotheram-Borus with funding from federal mental-health and drug-abuse agencies. Many of the young people in this study reported mental-health problems (suicidality), drug use, and other problems—dangerous sexual behavior, running away, and extremely sex-atypical behavior and appearance. Again, investigators stated that there was "no evidence that the agency attracts primarily troubled youth."[15]

Being gay, young, and *troubled* had thus been intrinsically, even purposefully, linked. The linkage made grant proposals and justifications for increased educational and mental-health services an easier sell. Indeed, according to one review, topics about gay youth most frequently addressed in published research during this time were physical-health concerns such as STDs, counseling and mental health, risky behavior, (poor) school performance, and (no) family support.[16]

As a result, mental-health advocates became increasingly sensitized to the needs of these distressed teenagers. Research data were employed as arguments for the inclusion of gay teens in the professional deliberations and services of physicians, therapists, and educators.[17] One clinician, Alan Malyon, exhorted mental-health professionals to help gay youths overcome their "impoverished socialization" so that they can adapt "to a stigmatized identity [that] is inherently problematic."[18] Similarly, sexologist Eli Coleman argued that therapists should "assist homosexual individuals to recognize and accept their sexual identity, improve interpersonal and social functioning, and value and integrate this identity while living in a predominately heterosexual society."[19]

These advocates spotlighted the difficulties of being young and gay. This image became (perhaps) unwittingly cemented during the first national symposium on gay and lesbian youth. Held in 1986 in Minneapolis, the conference signaled that the field of gay adolescence was coming into its own. The purpose of the gathering, according to its organizer, Gary Remafedi, was to address the medical, psychological, and social needs of gay youths and to form a national network of services for them. Workshop presenters included a parent, a minister, a state senator, a lawyer, a physician, a health educator, a youth worker, a social worker, a clinician, an activist, and a sociologist. There was no developmental psychologist, no specialist in adolescent development and few non–applied scientists. Not surprisingly, the vast majority of formal presentations and workshops focused on the "challenges" faced by gay teens, including homelessness, peer rejection, prostitution, chemical abuse, mental-health dysfunction, STDs, AIDS, and the need for medical services and various prevention and intervention strategies. I attended the conference as an observer.[20]

A review of the literature that came out of this era reveals that, in general, little of the research was published in peer-reviewed, top-tier social science journals. In addition, these early findings were rarely incorporated into mainstream scholarship on adolescents or cited in textbooks on adolescent development. Although reasons for this exclusion and the separation of gay teens from the field of adolescent development are a matter of debate, the following are plausible:

1. Relatively few research designs met the stringent methodological requirements of scholarly research, particularly with regard to population recruitment and research instruments.
2. The belief, held by perhaps a majority of scholars, that gayness did not exist as a stable entity during adolescence (rather, it was

seen as experimental, a phase, a curiosity) precluded journal editors from publishing research that was submitted.

3. Investigators did not submit their reports to top-tier journals because they did not believe their research would be treated seriously and objectively.

4. Most investigators were medical and clinical personnel and naturally submitted their work to specialty journals. This resulted in many scholars of adolescence being unaware of existing research.

5. Much of the best research went unpublished because it was conducted by doctoral students who either did not want to be tainted by the gay label or who were intent on becoming clinicians and thus were less interested in publishing their research findings.

In defense of mainstream adolescent scholarship and its failure to be inclusive, generally accepted scientific standards could not easily ignore the fact that all early gay-youth investigations were based on flawed research designs and included small or biased samples of those who sought the services of mental-health or social-support agencies. In defense of these early researchers, they must have been so pleased to have access to any gay teens that any slippage in standards for methodological rigor seemed relatively inconsequential; to provide any information on this nearly invisible population was an admirable and satisfying accomplishment. Policy-oriented exhortations on the treatment needs of gay youth and recommendations for physical- and mental-health guidelines for practitioners raised the consciousness of many. Whether the findings of these researchers could be generalized to the far larger number of "unmarked," non–gay-identified adolescents with same-sex attractions who did not volunteer for research was not seriously considered.

As I read this literature in the late 1980s, I couldn't ignore my skepticism. How typical were these young people? How could inferences be drawn about gay development from those most likely to be suffering physically, psychologically, and socially? From a purely scientific perspective, the investigations were methodologically flawed because they included only a very small number of non-representative lesbians, bisexuals, and gay males from crisis centers, runaway shelters, support groups, and collegiate activist groups.[21] Despite the assurances of the front-line researchers and advocacy warriors, how could I legitimately consider knowledge about these self-referred teens in distress to be typical? Worse yet, I could not suppress a lingering reservation: maybe the information was actually counterproductive.

Still, what we might call the "first wave" of gay youth studies in the 1970s and 1980s did result in some useful developments:

- The first research specifications of gay youth are provided in 1972.
- The New York City Institute for the Protection of Lesbian and Gay Youth opens in 1979.
- Small-scale studies on the lives of "unusual" gay youth escalate in the late 1980s.
- Mental-health providers and educators use this research to advocate for sensitivity to the plight of gay teens.
- The 1986 National Symposium on Gay and Lesbian Youth in Minneapolis is held, formally recognizing the existence of gay youth.

The 1980s and 1990s: Suicidal Script

By the 1980s we knew that gay teens existed. Journal articles about them increased dramatically, from several in the 1970s to nearly 40 in the 1980s to over 120 in the 1990s.[22] Although special issues of journals devoted to gay youth were published in the late 1980s,[23] mainstream social science journals lagged far behind. The first adolescent journal that dedicated an issue to gay youth was published in 1994.[24]

The flagship journal of the Society for Research on Adolescence published its first *article* on gay youth in 1998.[25]

Many of the earlier investigators of the 1980s and 1990s remained obliged to social or mental-health agencies for recruitment. Small-scale qualitative studies were also common—for example, only 50 gay and lesbian teenagers took part in a California study and 25 lesbians in a Toronto project.[26] Yet things were beginning to change. Groups of investigators attempted to address the problem of bias in study samples by administering surveys to school-based populations in Vermont, Massachusetts, and Minnesota.[27] They appeared to be unaware, however, that enlisting research participants in public schools does not necessarily guarantee that a representative, or even diverse, sample of teens with same-sex attractions would be willing to check the socially stigmatized "gay" identity box on a questionnaire. Indeed, researcher Theo Sandfort argued that no sample could truly be representative because the base characteristics of what constitutes homosexuality is unknown.[28] In addition, many factors influence decisions about whether to expose oneself. A young woman, for example, growing up in the Midwest or South is less likely than an adolescent of either coast to risk labeling herself lesbian.[29]

In reality, contemporary teenagers who willingly identify as gay on school-based questionnaires are not so different from the young gay subjects of the 1980s—the "out," visible, early identifying, help-seeking teens. Although no published study has to my knowledge directly compared very "out" students to those who are more discreet, school-based surveys usually elicit a gay identification response from only a small fraction (1–2 percent) of the total adolescent population completing the survey. This proportion is considerably below population estimates of those who have same-sex attractions. Thus, investigators who argue that they have a representative sample of gay teenagers because they recruited their sample from public high schools may have only drawn the same participants as those studied in earlier investigations of support-group youth.[30]

Another group of investigators of the 1980s and 1990s implemented research designs more typical of the social sciences. They did so primarily by recruiting young people from a variety of venues. As a result, ethnically diverse gay teens, young lesbians, bisexuals, and gay people from various countries (England, France, Mexico, Brazil, Australia, Sweden) were thus made visible. Gay adolescents could be found in routine public settings and at community picnics, collegiate meetings, friendship networks, and activist conferences. Several of these large-scale surveys focused less on mental-health problems and psychosocial stressors and more on typical cultural and developmental milestones. They determined that gay adolescents have sexual attractions, sexual experiences, disclosures to friends and parents, and committed romantic relationships.[31]

I emphasize survey population sources so much because I believe they are important. One piece of evidence that this is so is provided by Theo Sandfort, who compared *adult* gay men in the Netherlands drawn from a random telephone survey to a group drawn from gay magazine readership and membership in gay organizations. The former were more religious, less educated, more politically conservative, more likely to be in a romantic relationship (that lasted longer), and less sexually promiscuous. He concluded that we know little about same-sex-attracted individuals "who are not linked, either superficially or strongly, to the gay world."[32]

Unfortunately, little is known about young people who, for unidentified reasons, self-select out of research. Perhaps they feel less positive about their sexuality and are loath to embrace a socially ostracized identity label. This does not necessarily imply, however, that they are thus less mentally well—only that they followed different developmental trajectories from others of their peers.

Perhaps their refusal to identify themselves reflects their belief that they aren't "gay youth," but a youth who happens to be gay. In this they'd agree with *Queer Eye for the Straight Guy* designer Thom Filicia, who said, "You know what, I *am* gay, but my sexuality has never been my defining quality. It's just a fact. My life is defined by my friends and by my interests, and I happen to be passionate about good design."[33] They object to being forced into a sexually laden identity category—being defined solely or primarily by their sexuality—being dehumanized. They think of themselves simply as *teenagers*, and they want to be accepted as such.

These gay teens also may choose not to participate in surveys for the same reasons teens don't volunteer for other scientific sexuality studies. They're less sexually experienced. They hold traditional sexual attitudes and beliefs. They have lower levels of sexual sensation-seeking or a lower libido. They're more likely to self-monitor their expressive behavior, including their sexuality.[34] If any one of these is true—and this is highly likely given their fundamental status as normal adolescents—then professionals' gay youth samples are distorted.

Critical caution is thus in order when evaluating the scientific merit of the published research cited in this book. Critiques of existing research in the 1980s and 1990s raised a number of concerns, both theoretical and methodological.[35] Among the most pertinent:

- an overreliance on recollections from gay adults on their adolescence rather than evidence on how gay adolescents "experience their lives as they are living them, rather than as they are *remembered*"
- narrow focus of research on the dramatic, such as sex-atypical behavior and parental rejection, rather than on the normative
- failure to track the same individuals over time to better understand developmental processes
- a concentration on what goes wrong in the lives of gay youth rather than the "features associated with the capacity to remain resilient when confronted by adverse life circumstances"
- the realization that to understand gay adolescents you must first understand adolescence in general (an insight that remains largely ignored even today)

During these years I read the published empirical research, I considered the wisdom of the advice literature, and I listened to experts supposedly "in the know" about gay youth. Then I contrasted these findings with the responses of young people to my survey questionnaires and my own interactions with large numbers of young people with same-sex attractions, and I began to have doubts. What exactly were we professionals doing? Were same-sex-attracted adolescents all so humorless and screwed up? Maybe they had adapted to their biology and their heterocentric culture. Maybe they were *healthy*. Maybe we adults were wrong.

Without minimizing the experiences of those in distress, I wanted to suggest that there was another side to being young and gay. Not all such adolescents were suicidal. I wanted to argue against a problem-centered approach and for a perspective that celebrates the promise and diversity of gay teens. This was the message I most wanted our young people to hear and believe. If they listened to us experts, I feared they'd be apt to give up, reach the conclusion that their life was inevitably distraught, perhaps even eventually kill themselves. Surely a better alternative existed.[36]

Other researchers shared my doubts and had the data to prove it. Most prophetic was a small sample of 37 African American gay and bisexual males. Most did not identify as gay, yet they were healthy, well-adjusted, and stable in their social functioning, with no need for counseling. They did not want their sexuality to be made public or for family members to know that they were gay. Yet—perhaps most surprisingly—they did not regret their sexuality, and were even proud of it.[37] The young men in this study could be said to be the harbinger of the next wave of research subjects.

The "second wave" of gay-youth study in the 1980s and 1990s, however, was not without its positive developments. It included:

- a dramatic expansion of research articles with a wider range of sample recruitment
- the publication of special issues of professional journals devoted to gay youth

- the launching of large-scale investigations of gay youth
- recognition that research participants might not be representative of the larger population of same-sex-attracted adolescents
- the publication of the first methodological critiques of extant gay-youth research

The Present: Resilience

By the beginning of the new century, a number of innovations regarding the study of gay adolescents were in the works. Perhaps most fundamentally, the definition of who counted as a "gay" adolescent was expanded. The first inkling that this issue might be critical was provided by AIDS researchers. They realized early in the pandemic that targeting at-risk individuals based on sexual *behavior* (e.g., men who have sex with men) was of far greater importance than targeting at-risk groups based on sexual *identity* or labels (e.g., "gay" or "bisexual" men). This was especially true among African Americans and Latinos, who were less likely than whites to embrace a socially stigmatized label to describe their same-sex behavior.[38] Perhaps, too, limiting inclusion in research and AIDS outreach programs to those who identified as "gay" excluded many young men who had only some, not all, of the characteristics of "gay youth." The potential consequences of such exclusion in the AIDS era were not known, but assumed to be profound.

A more inclusive definition was also valuable in research with young women. During their young-adult years, the majority of college-aged, same-sex-attracted women shift sexual identities, sometimes multiple times.[39] This fluidity in sexual identification necessarily discredits traditional means of identifying who should be included as lesbian or bisexual. Only by assessing the relative strength of same- versus opposite-sex physical and romantic interests can young women's future sexual lives be predicted.

Thus, when seeking young women to interview for my latest research, I relied not on an identity label ("lesbians and bisexuals") but on descriptions of attractions ("If you have physical, romantic, or sexual attractions to other women"). This more inclusive recruitment strategy I hoped would result in my attracting a range of women, who would have various histories of same-sex attractions and behaviors, and would not exclude young women who might decline to identify as lesbian or bisexual but who nevertheless acknowledge a same-sex sexuality.

When should one recruit by sexual identity labels and when by sexual orientation or behavior? It depends on the research question. If, for example, the question concerns discrimination or victimization, sexual labels might be quite germane because a gay identity often elicits these reactions. However, if the question concerns behavioral outcomes such as pregnancy, sexually transmitted infection, or virginity status, then identity labels are of little use; sexual behavior is of far greater relevance. If one wishes to understand the development of cognitive performance, brain structure, and career selection, then the persistence of and preferred object of sexual arousal, desire, and attractions (in other words, sexual orientation) is the variable of choice.

One real-world consequence illustrates these differences. Which of these domains of sexuality a young woman reveals to her parents might very well determine how they react. Consider the various aspects of her sexuality that a daughter can tell her mother.[40]

- An assumed-to-be universal statement of apparently little consequence: "Mom, I'm attracted to girls."
- A behavioral statement, more serious than the first, but still seemingly benign: "Mom, I'm dating girls."
- A behavioral statement that is likely to be frightening to parents because it defines homosexuality and reveals that their "little girl" is sexual: "Mom, I'm having sex with girls."
- A sexual identity statement with ostensibly lifelong repercussions and negative stereotypes: "Mom, I'm a lesbian."

Another advance researchers have made in the early years of the twenty-first century is that they are increasingly willing to use new recruitment strategies, especially the Internet. The Web gives teens who don't live in academic communities or urban areas access to much new information, including information on research projects. They might be more likely to volunteer for studies using the Internet because there is less risk of exposure. True, Internet recruitment has problems of its own. Only those with Internet access and those who are sufficiently computer savvy can participate. Does this result in an oversampling of geeks and an undersampling of jocks? It's also difficult to verify response accuracy. Is the respondent who claims to be thirteen years old really thirteen or a sixty-four-year-old posing as thirteen? Despite these problems, the Internet remains a powerful and useful tool, especially for accessing hidden populations, including those who, because of their socially stigmatized characteristics, fear the limelight.

Perhaps the most far-reaching Internet effort is a survey of "queer and questioning youth." The 2000 OutProud/Oasis survey was completed by 1,199 individuals from seventy-five countries, mostly English-speaking. Nearly 30 percent of these respondents were "out" only on the Internet. The vast majority, 85 percent, had never attended a gay support group. Traditional investigators using social service or community gay support groups would have missed most of these teenagers.[41] This ability of the Internet to access the hard to reach, including rural populations and those who do not currently identify as gay, was the primary reason a group of Australian researchers decided to use the Internet for their national report on "same-sex attracted young people."[42]

Researchers now also have the unique opportunity to use questions that probe aspects of same-sex sexuality among *all* respondents in several large-scale studies. The National Longitudinal Study of Adolescent Health ("Add Health" for short) asks about same-sex romantic attractions, sexual behavior with girls and boys, and sexual identity from straight to gay. This is done through the use of audio computer-aided self-interviews, which encourages honesty and anonymity. Researcher Stephen Russell points out that these measures and techniques likely capture a broad range of junior and senior high school students who have some degree of same-sex sexuality, most of whom don't identify as gay.[43]

The fact that Add Health follows the same students over time points out another present-day advance: researchers are attempting to understand the evolution of developmental processes during the life course. Although an early two-year longitudinal study was conducted in the late 1980s with recruits from the Hetrick-Martin Institute,[44] developments over the past several years have made follow-up research designs dramatically easier to carry out. For example, the most ambitious longitudinal study to date includes over 500 young gay people in what's known as "The Q & A Project." Researchers Tony D'Augelli and Arnie Grossman are probing the connections between verbal harassment and physical violence on mental health and the evolution of developmental milestones. These studies are possible because anonymity is now both available and, given the increasing destigmatization of same-sex sexuality, optional.

The most successful longitudinal project is probably Lisa Diamond's. It involves 89 young women, originally between the ages of sixteen and twenty-three years. Begun in 1995 with a ten-year follow-up interview being planned, 90 percent of the young women have stayed in the study.[45] What reasons does Diamond give for her success? As she told me:

> Persistence is the big one. I would use a lot of detective work to track folks down if their contact information did not pan out. The Internet sure helped. The young women were always real keen on staying involved because they really liked the project, too. Maybe it also helped that at the time I was a graduate student, close in age to them. So the distance between us, power-wise, is not as great as it is for some researcher/subject relationships, and maybe that helps.[46]

Research agendas are also becoming more diverse. Gay adolescent research has been de-ghettoized and has reached over to mainstream social science journals, textbooks, and public policy. Particular findings about gay youth are linked with basic, broader psychological issues such as female sexuality, developmental trajectories, and developmental and social processes. For the first time, a more normative, holistic, and healthy portrait of same-sex-attracted teenagers can be imagined. No longer are they solely portrayed "[as] though they do not exist or as objects of hate and bigotry."[47] Some scholars now admit that, perhaps despite great odds, some gay teens are actually quite resilient.

Thus, the following are present-day advances in research on gay adolescents:

- Population definitions of same-sex sexuality have been expanded beyond identity labels to incorporate behavioral measures.
- Novel recruitment strategies, especially the Internet and mainstream surveys, have been initiated.
- Longitudinal research designs have become more common.
- Diversification of research agendas now characterizes many investigations.

The Wave of the Future: Ordinary

The overall portrait of gay teenagers during the past thirty years has evolved from a population under siege to the possibility of resiliency. Pathos reigned when we simply let a select group of adolescents "tell their story." Limited to, and in response to, these troubled teens, of course researchers would have written a suicidal script. It is important to keep in mind, however, that an opposite result occurred when "overt homosexual" men told their stories in Evelyn Hooker's politically charged, policy-driven research published in the 1950s.[48] Hooker's finding that these men displayed "average adjustment" countered psychiatric malfeasance and diagnostic disorders that were supposedly inherent in being gay. Hooker pointed out in 1957 that sampling from therapy-attending populations amplified and overgeneralized stereotypes of maladjustment. You would have thought that gay youth researchers would have taken note of, and agreed with, this assertion.

Instead, they repeated the mistake. Researchers exploring gay youth fought the dragons of discrimination and sexual prejudice, but fell into the trap that Hooker had warned them of. I have little doubt that these scholars and mental-health professionals intended to help gay teens, not to show how pathetic young gay people's lives are. They wanted to promote intervention and prevention programs that would improve the physical and psychic health of gay youth. Unfortunately, the consequences of their approach, however unintended and unanticipated, turned out to be counterproductive, handicapping the field for decades thereafter.

More seriously, this approach affected young lives. One young man I interviewed in the 1990s questioned whether he should or could participate in my research. "I don't think I'm gay," he said to me. "I haven't tried to kill myself yet." When I showed myself unable to hide my surprise at his words, he added, "Well, I've read so much about gay youth suicide that I thought that was a rite of passage." If the overwhelming message we gave young people who were considering whether to disclose their sexuality was "Be Prepared to Die," would you come out? Would the acceptance of your sexuality by yourself or others increase or decrease? Would you be proud or ashamed of your sexuality?

The investigators who published these negative findings knew what they were doing. They were aware of their sample limitations, that they had recruited those disproportionately at risk for negative health outcomes and risk behaviors. Yet few attempted to correct this portrait of the suffering gay adolescent.[49] Rather, follow the money trail—grants—to explicitly address what was *wrong*, not what was right about their lives.[50] Nevertheless, this research resulted in some positive outcomes. A number of political, social, and educational organizations dedicated to bettering the lives of gay teenagers were founded. Once those organizations were in place, additional data were needed to support their explicit missions: Reduce antigay violence and discrimination. Educate mental-health professionals about the gay teens in their midst. Enter hetero-normative settings (such as the public school system) to alert the administration, faculty, and peers about the gay young people in their midst and how damaging their insensitive and barbaric behavior could be. Authenticate and hence address the possibility of suicide among those struggling with their same-sex sexuality.

In this kind of environment, the ability of teenagers with same-sex attractions to withstand and adapt to oppression and its effects went unnoticed, unrecorded, and unexplained. Yet it is clear to me that many youth who happen to have same-sex attractions live their lives in much the same way that those with heterosexual attractions do. They go to football games, try out for cheerleader, run for Student Council, argue with their parents, and wonder what to wear. Somehow we missed this; but we won't in the future if we listen to their lives.

4

Models or Trajectories?

After the creation of gay youth during the 1970s and 1980s, clinicians developed idealized models of how one becomes gay. Adolescence turned out to be a critical time in what was seen as a universal, linear process. Convenient, easy-to-remember stages were proposed by which one could trace the transition from childhood recognition of same-sex attractions to adolescent acceptance of a gay identity to young-adult commitment to and integration of a gay identity.

These "coming-out" or "sexual identity" models began as a trickle, eventually became a tidal wave, and have not yet subsided. By my conservative estimate, over two dozen experts have created separate models of sexual identity development. All have been seduced by the intuitive appeal of conceiving of development as a simple, lockstep formulation; some by the possibility of fame.[1] Despite prolific claims to exceptionality, in nearly all constructions of these "master" narratives, the shift from "thinking" gay to "doing" gay to "being" gay occurs in a fairly uniform fashion. One is said to move from a private same-sex sexuality (at times unknown to oneself) to a public sexuality fully integrated into one's sense of self. Gay people, first, are supposed to recognize that they are different; then they realize that this difference might be linked to their sexuality. At that point they give a name to it, publicize their sexual status to others, and integrate their same-sex sexuality into their sense of self. Easy, clear, and obvious.

These models remain at least as popular today as they were when they were first proposed three decades ago—and there is no end in sight. Additional, "new" versions continue to appear. Recently promised are a *new* "inclusive model of lesbian identity assumption," a *new* "social identity perspective," a *new* "inclusive model of sexual minority formation," and a *new* "multidimensional process."[2]

Where do these sexual identity models come from? Although they grow out of various theoretical orientations, their ultimate, though seldom acknowledged, historic and theoretical source is Erik Erikson, the "father of identity development."

Erikson and Identity Development

According to psychoanalyst Erik Erikson, the unique developmental task of adolescence is to solidify a personal identity.[3] Although one's identity begins to evolve at infancy and continues to do so throughout the life course, adolescence is the critical time for its development. The task involves expanding one's perception of self-sameness and feeling the continuity of one's existence in time and space. It is also critical that others recognize this sameness and continuity. Forming an identity is neither static nor immutable; it allows teens to know where they've been and where they're going.

The ultimate goal is to emerge at the end of adolescence with a firm sense of a functioning whole. The teenager may find the process pleasurable, even if the culture disapproves or condemns the outcome (a negative identity), because in identity formation an adolescent gains "an increased sense of inner unity, with an increase of good judgment, and an increase in the capacity 'to do well' according to his own standards and to the standards of those who are significant to him."[4]

Given the cultural context and the time when Erikson was writing (the 1950s and 1960s), developing a *positive* individual or group identity that coalesced around sexual status was not in anyone's inventory of possibilities. If adolescents felt marginalized because of their particular identity process, they might turn away from normative ideals toward a *negative* identity that would frustrate and alienate their parents. One such negative identity is a homosexual identity, a rebellion against parental values and an acceptance of "all those identifications and roles which, at critical stages of development, had been presented to them as most undesirable or dangerous and yet also as most real."[5] To Erikson, homosexuality is a negative, desperate attempt to regain mastery when routes toward positive identity appear unachievable. It is easier for a person to be sure of something, even if that something is as devalued as homosexuality, than to suffer a confused identity.[6]

The Cass Sexual Identity Model

The six-stage development model of Vivienne Cass has become, by near unanimous acclaim, the standard bearer of homosexual identity models.[7] Unlike many of her peers, Cass continues to refine and expand the model she first proposed during her predoctoral days in the late 1970s. Sexual identity, according to Cass, is a universal developmental process that proceeds in a predetermined temporal sequence of six stages (from the following list, note that identity diffusion or foreclosure is to be avoided, while testing out one's identity and advancing toward identity synthesis is to be encouraged):[8]

   1. Identity confusion. Stage 1 begins when an individual recognizes that his or her sexual feelings, actions, or thoughts could be labeled homosexual and ends with the declaration to oneself either "No, I'm not" (identity foreclosure) or "Yes, I am" (identity exploration). Previous sexual identities are questioned, but not rejected. Emotional tension, bewilderment, and anxiety are common at this stage.

2. *Identity comparison.* In Stage 2, an individual compares his or her sexual feelings with those of others and tentatively accepts them: "I might be." The stage ends with an acknowledgement of identity: "I probably am." Through self-examination and the feedback of others, the individual evaluates this possibility as desirable (true sense of self), too costly (alienation from family and friends), or a temporary aberration (bisexual, a special case of desire).

3. *Identity tolerance.* Stage 3 begins with a tentative belief ("I likely am") and ends with certainty, albeit without full acceptance ("I am, but I don't want to be"). The individual gains greater clarity about how this identity affects other domains of the self. Initial contacts with other homosexuals are made, and well-trusted heterosexuals are informed. These experiences lead the individual either to devalue or minimize contact with other homosexuals, or to deepen acceptance and commitment to a homosexual status.

4. *Identity acceptance.* Stage 4 individuals have a clearer and more positive image of themselves as homosexual: "It's okay that I'm gay." Comfortable among other homosexuals, those at this stage make selective disclosures to others, although passing as straight (foreclosure) may occur. Discrepancies between positive reactions when among gays and negative reactions when among heterosexuals lead to Stage 5.

5. *Identity pride.* Incongruity between the homosexual and heterosexual worlds propels Stage 5. The universe is dichotomized into the gay (source of pride) and the not-gay (source of anger): "I'm gay and proud of it." The inevitable confrontations inspire a preference for associations with like-minded people.

6. *Identity synthesis.* The private and the public homosexual selves merge in Stage 6. An integrated sense of self as homosexual with other aspects of the self is achieved. Being homosexual is an important but not exclusive aspect of the self: "I'm a poet who is gay, not a gay poet." The person is at peace, feels self-actualized and not defensive, and has positive interactions with those who are not gay.

OBJECTIONS

Given that multistage models of homosexuality describe an inherent unfolding of development, then the various stages should be observable, verifiable, and uniform across time and space. Gay identification is thus the same for all, and with a discernible beginning and end. Criticism of these models arose almost as soon as the first one was published. The criticisms have been broad and deep, at times vitriolic, and usually quite penetrating.[9] On the positive side of the ledger, few would deny that gay adolescence was brought to mainstream scholarly attention in large part because of sexual identity models. Thus, their contribution cannot be easily dismissed. More controversial is whether this contribution neutralizes the serious negative consequences the models impose on an understanding of adolescent same-sex sexuality.

Those who have posited models have sometimes recognized that their stages might not mirror absolute fact. Clinician Eli Coleman was perhaps most forthcoming on this score.[10] He warned that his sequence of stages does not exactly fit reality because of the complexity and diversity of the gay population. Some people are not exclusively gay. Some do not achieve an integrated identity. Some remain developmentally static. People's lives are far more chaotic, fluid, and complex than any simple model might suggest.

Richard Troiden proposed an admittedly idealized model to enable clinicians to meet the needs of their lesbian and gay patients.[11]

The stages of his model are merely benchmarks against which to describe and test various hypotheses. More spiral than linear, Troiden's model suggests that individuals move back and forth between stages and that not all will experience all stages or substages. Development is thus moderated by both external factors (such as heterocentrism and sexual prejudice) and internal factors (such as one's internalized homophobia and character strengths). Even Vivienne Cass cautioned that her model "is not intended that it should be true in all respects for all people since individuals and situations are inherently complex." Variations occur in rate of progression, paths taken, coping strategies available within each stage, and the final state achieved.[12]

Given these reservations, even from those who have put forward the models, it is somewhat surprising that anyone would actually use them. Moreover, these theoretical objections have been joined by critics of the models who simply ask the straightforward question "Are they true?"—that is, do the lives of same-sex-attracted individuals follow sexual identity models? After all, to be useful the models must reflect real life and not merely scientific hypotheses.

The fact is, the empirical base for these models is extraordinarily scant. One scholar noted of the models that people appear to be wedged or "forced into stages, rather than stages made to fit people's situations."[13] Perhaps the models survive because they appear intuitively obvious, even in the face of apparent disconfirming evidence.

One criticism, substantially supported, is that sexual identity models are particularly insensitive to cohort, gender, and ethnicity. Feminist scholars have not been subtle in their critiques. They charge that stage models are an imposition of dominant white male development posturing as normative and unfairly extrapolated to female development. Clinician Laura Brown considered the mere attempt to impose uniformity on the creative chaos of female lives to be repugnant.[14] Others see little evidence for an "essential lesbian self, no set of uniquely lesbian experiences that can be discovered through introspection."[15] Young women, regardless of their orientation, often claim some degree of same-sex attraction, question their identity, reject identity labels altogether or are multi-identified, and change labels over time.[16] This may be because of the way girls are socialized—into a broad, exploratory range of behavioral and emotional intimacies that result in a gradual, fluid, and ambiguous identity development, lacking rank order or privileged aspects of identity. Girls' development might thus be quite different from boys' coming to terms with their same-sex sexuality.[17]

Other scholars agree, raising doubts that a linear model pertains to women. Paula Rodríguez Rust eschewed developmental sexual identity stages altogether in favor of representing young women's lives in terms of fluidity. Some young women, even lesbian-identified ones, have sex with men without disturbing their sense of sexuality. Or they have sex with men during periods of doubt and questioning. Variation and fluidity are the rule, not the exception. Any clearly demarcated (artificial) boundaries between lesbians, bisexuals, and other women fail to capture the essence of their lives.[18]

Historian Lillian Faderman allows that some older "homosexual females" might have conformed to the models.[19] They identified as lesbian late in life, often by becoming involved in the feminist movement; feminism led them to critically evaluate social norms that dictated heterosexuality. Unlike these women, who "became" lesbian after many years of heterosexual relationships and marriage, today's young lesbians traverse a path based more on relational than political reasons.[20]

Others have suggested that coming-out models appear more applicable to some and not other cohorts. Perhaps those who entered adolescence during the 1960s and 1970s, when the models were first proposed, followed the models.[21] Counseling youth over several decades convinced John Gonsiorek that contemporary young people experience a truncated or more rapid identity development process, coming out to others while still in their teens. Their lives do not faithfully mirror the stages in the published literature. For example, contemporary young men were more likely than their older gay brothers to identify as gay prior to having sex with another male. These differences are not inconsequential. Gay men who have sex with other males before identifying as gay had higher levels of internalized homophobia, more heterosexual sex and relationships, and more male sex partners.[22]

A third criticism, that the prevailing assumptions of sexual identity models are ethnocentric, notes that "progress" is measured in terms of movement along a white, majority continuum. African American, Latino, Asian American, and Native American Indian young people are profoundly influenced by specific cultural, class, and historic contexts.[23] In their communities, sexual identity can be strategic and situational, "continually being negotiated and renegotiated in response to life events and historical/social forces."[24] The prospect of identity fluidity is not one easily accommodated in most sexual identity models. Yet for many ethnic-minority teens, identity choices are rarely cemented but must remain open to negotiation. Can I live openly as gay in my ethnic community and maintain my ethnic heritage in the gay community? Do these identity terms carry extra ramifications to my immediate and extended family members? How can I cope with the racism embedded in gay communities?[25]

Research supports these criticisms. Levels of self-acceptance and "outness" among African American young men are reflected in whether they are in a same-sex romantic relationship with a white or a black man. If they are dating a white man, their primary allegiance tends to be with the gay rather than the black community, and as a result they experience less family and ethnic community support. If they are dating a black man, they tend to feel alienated from the gay community, but more connected to their ethnic heritage.[26] Additionally, an underground "down low" (DL) culture exists among contemporary African American young men, which is regressive according to traditional sexual identity models but reflects a novel means of integrating same-sex sexuality within an African American identity. The DL culture is comprised of black men who maintain strict hypermasculine behavior, a heterosexual identity, heterosexual relationships, and same-sex behavior. It is a movement that actively defies, even ridicules, the gay label, which is interpreted as being more about femme or sissy men than about same-sex behavior. Fearing that they will "let down the whole black community, black women, black history, black pride," these men consciously elect to conceal their same-sex longings from those not in the scene.[27]

A study I did with Eric Dubé found marked ethnic-group differences among young men in the timing and sequence of developmental milestones.[28] For example:

- Latinos were early and Asian Americans late in awareness of their same-sex attractions.
- Many African Americans but few Asian Americans had gay sex before identifying as gay.
- Asian Americans engaged in gay sex at a later age.
- African Americans and whites were more likely than Asian Americans and Latinos to have sex with females.
- African Americans and Asian Americans were least likely to be out to others, especially to family members.

One might be tempted to interpret these results as meaning that certain ethnic groups are apt to be more identity-integrated and thus healthier than others. This would be a serious miscalculation. The groups did not differ in internalized homophobia. In another study, Japanese Americans seldom reached the final stages of identity integration.[29] Neglected was the fact that Japanese culture provides few opportunities for individuals to synthesize their sexual identity through a visible, gay presentation of self or to establish a sense of gay identity. Coming out to others or engaging in political activism might not be realistic indicators of sexual identity formation within this cultural context.

YOUNG LIVES

Another, particularly damning, objection to the sexual identity models comes from individuals themselves. When carefully examined, few appear to follow proposed sequences.

Clinician Joan Sophie illustrated this fact in the 1980s in her interviews with women.[30] To cite just three examples:

- Nan lived an exclusively lesbian lifestyle for thirteen years with two romantic relationships of three and ten years' duration, but she never identified as lesbian. She began dating men because she wanted social approval and heterosexual privileges. She reported no sexual label.
- Amy became a gay activist in college, but then realized she was bisexual because she fell in love with her best (gay) male friend. She dated a few men before deciding that her sexuality did not have to be consistent with her politics.
- Hi became intimate with a boy in high school and lived with him for six years, until age twenty-one. During this time she became involved in a passionate female relationship, which caused her to question her heterosexuality. Association with lesbian groups led her to a period of identity exploration. She eventually labeled herself lesbian, but then decided that labels were too limiting. Sexuality was of such low priority to Hi that she ultimately decided that no label was best.

Similarly, most of the young men I interviewed also failed to follow the strictures of sexual identity models.[31] Although the average age at which they reached various milestones appeared to match those suggested by the coming-out models, the sequence these young

Table 4.1 Age for reaching developmental milestones: Ian, Matt, and Sean

	Same-sex attractions	Possibly gay	Label self	Associate with gays	Romantic relationship
Ian	5	12	18	18	15
Matt	10	10	9	18+	18+
Sean	16	16	18	13	18
Mean age	10.3	12.7	15.0	16.3	17.0

men followed tells a very different story. Table 4.1 presents the mean ages of reaching developmental milestones for three of these young men. Their stories follow.

- Ian recalled same-sex attractions as among his earliest memories, but his sexual development "got arrested" until the onset of puberty, when he realized that his feelings were homosexual. He suppressed this knowledge from himself until he fell madly in love with his best friend, his first true love affair. This did not necessarily mean to him that he was gay or that he wanted to associate with gay people. These realizations had to wait until he entered college.
- In response to being called "fag," Matt understood that he must be gay, and so he labeled himself as such at age nine. It was only afterward that he recognized that his thoughts and feelings were homoerotic. Although now eighteen, Matt has not fallen in love with a man, nor has he disclosed his sexuality to others.
- Sean began hanging out with his gay brother and friends in eighth grade. This led to a sexual experience, which he wanted and which was his first memory of having same-sex attractions and feelings. Once he fell in love during his freshman year of college, he labeled himself gay.

In short, the lives of many, if not most, young women and men do not fit tidily into these "master narratives."[32] Even if most models are inherently male-centric, research suggests that they even fail to characterize the lives of current cohorts of young men with same-sex attractions.[33] Of the many young people I interviewed, only 2 percent of the young men, and none of the young women, adhered to the published sexual identity models.

SEXUAL IDENTITY MODELS RECONSIDERED

Sexual identity models helped establish gay adolescence as a field of scholarship and suggested clinical and policy applications. Their usefulness, however, has been compromised because they have proven to be incapable of adequately characterizing the dynamic lives of contemporary young people. Unless a sexual identity model explicitly rejects universalism and includes contextual, cultural, and historic considerations, it is doomed as an obsolete relic of a time when development was perceived as predetermined and universal. If models were to follow these strictures, however, what would be left worth keeping? Within a given person's life, do such well-defined starting and ending points in the search for identity exist? Don't individual paths, as one writer put it, "run parallel, diverge, intersect, and perhaps merge at a later point?"[34] The concept of separate stages inherently places brackets around something that can't be bracketed. An individual's life is more than a category, and is always in a state of flux and self-discovery. Life is dynamic, in perpetual reinvention rather than sitting at a concluding point.[35]

If sexual identity models are to have a future, several problems must be addressed. First, they usually assume a bivariate typology. Gay or straight. Take your pick. But don't choose bisexual, or unlabeled, or queerboi. Yet, even if we accept just two choices, has any attention ever been paid to the heterosexual portion of the bimodal distribution? Where are the models of heterosexual sexual identity? How does an adolescent come to adopt a heterosexual sexual identity? Do heterosexuals even have a sexual identity? If not, why not? Shouldn't they also struggle and evolve? If they don't have to, then needing to progress through stages to achieve a sexual identity makes one inherently deviant. What would happen if the stigma attached to homosexuality is greatly reduced or disappears? Does a sexual identity only exist in the presence of stigma toward unorthodox sexualities? To accept the validity of models of development for gay people only implies a succumbing to heterosexual values, norms, and definitions of reality.[36]

Another, related problem is that some heterosexuals do question their sexual orientation and consciously assume a sexual identity.[37] Where is their sexual identity model? Why are they questioning? Are we to conclude that heterosexuals who question their identity are by definition unhealthy?

Sexual identity models are easily faulted for oversimplifying a complex, evolving process. It is erroneous to assume that one model can apply to all, without regard to gender, background, cohort, ethnicity, or empirical validation. The failure of these attempts at modeling was inevitable. One critic charged these constructs as being "frameworks superimposed on phenomena by researchers" and that they "may be real only for their inventors."[38]

Alternatives, which reflect the diverse, unpredictable, and ever-changing lives of contemporary teens, are few. One, which I have argued for, is a *differential developmental trajectories* perspective.

Differential Developmental Trajectories

So little is known about the development of same-sex-attracted individuals that I believe it is irresponsible to propose a comprehensive theory. Rather, I lay out what might be called a "differential developmental trajectories" framework.

Differential refers to the variability inherent within and across individuals.
Developmental signifies the milestones and processes that occur across the life course.

Trajectories indicates the probabilistic individual pathways that occur through time and space.[39]

This framework retains features true to the real-life experiences of adolescents, including the notion of milestones, transitional incidents, fluidity, and positive development. A basic assumption is that sexuality is a valid context for adolescent development—for all adolescents, regardless of sexual orientation.

This framework discards the following three antiquated assumptions:

1. Life progresses along an orderly series of idealized sequential stages.
2. The complexity and diversity of developmental processes that shape lives need not be considered.
3. Young lives can be understood from research based on a population of highly selective adolescents (e.g., those who identify themselves as gay).

The differential developmental trajectories perspective of development takes into account what is and is not known about the lives of same-sex-attracted teens. For example, we know the age at which same-sex attractions first emerge, but little about their content, intensity, fluidity, or motivational influence; nor do we know how these sexual thoughts, fantasies, and attractions are experienced and interpreted. In addition, we know when young people first have sex with a partner, but little about what constitutes a sex partner or a sex act, how conflicting motivations for and against sexual activities are negotiated, and the various meanings and repercussions of sexual experience. And we know when first self-labeling as gay or bisexual occurs, but little about the reasons for and against self-labeling, whether alternative identities are considered, how bisexuality and gayness interact, and whether claiming a sexual identity is healthy.

To address these issues, I propose four basic tenets:[40]

1. Same-sex-attracted teenagers are similar to all other adolescents in their developmental trajectories. All are subject to the same biological, psychological, and social influences. To focus exclusively on the consequences of homoeroticism runs the danger of misattributing normal adolescent experiences to sexual orientation.

2. Same-sex-attracted teenagers are dissimilar from heterosexual adolescents in their developmental trajectories. Perhaps due to a unique, biologically mediated constitution and cultural heterocentrism (the latter especially manifested in negativity toward sex-atypical behavior, temperament, and interests), same-sex-attracted young people's psychological development is different from that of heterosexuals.

3. Same-sex-attracted teenagers vary among themselves in their developmental trajectories, and this can be similar to the ways in which heterosexual teens vary among themselves. The interaction of sexuality with gender, ethnicity, geography, socioeconomic status, and cohort results in distinctive trajectories among teens. It is imprudent to characterize same-sex desire as a monolith—a single entity with similar developmental trajectories and outcomes.

4. The developmental trajectory of a given person is similar to that of no other person who has ever lived. Given the profound diversity inherent in individual lives, general descriptions of group-mean differences and similarities may be irrelevant when applied to a specific individual.

ADOLESCENTS ARE ADOLESCENTS

The first tenet, that same-sex-attracted adolescents are, first and foremost, fundamentally adolescents and thus are similar to all other teens in developmentally significant ways, might appear so self-evident as to require little notation. Nevertheless, this perspective is often lost in portraits of their lives. Adolescents live within precise historic and cultural contexts and within basic biological systems and constraints. During childhood, adolescence, and eventual adulthood, they experience and negotiate age-appropriate developmental transitions and milestones. Although it is true that individual genetics vary and that societal influences are to some degree person specific, most basic developmental characteristics and processes are shared by most adolescents.

Same-sex-attracted teenagers are, in general, indistinguishable from other teens neurologically, anatomically, and chemically. They achieve their full height and genital maturity during puberty, develop novel ways of thinking, and accumulate knowledge just as other young people do. Also like other teens, they must negotiate parental and peer relationships. Teens of all sexualities think about and explore arenas of sexual and emotional intimacy. They hope to find a friend, to find a date, and to meet others "just like me." No sexual-orientation differences have been found in the chemistry of love, self-esteem level, feelings of mastery, perceived stress, availability of support, and number of romantic relationships.[41] Regardless of sexual orientation, young adults consider their educational and occupational future, develop a system of ethical values and conduct, and want the freedom to be themselves.

Same-sex-attracted adolescents, compared to their heterosexual peers, are said to have higher rates of difficulty and pain in their lives, including suicide and depression. To connect suicide to sexual prejudice is tempting, but this overlooks the impact of characteristics that place all young people, regardless of sexuality, at risk,[42] including such things as difficulty negotiating peer social relations, living in a dysfunctional family with little concomitant hope for support or understanding, having a mental illness, abusing substances, and witnessing others attempt suicide.[43] Rarely is sexuality per se the cause of suicide. If we want to know which homoerotic teens are most at risk for suicide, we should assess issues that negatively affect all teens.

SOME DISTINCTIONS

Same-sex-oriented teens may vary from heterosexual peers because of their biological constitution and socialization experiences. The extent to which this may be true and, if true, how developmentally significant it may be is a matter of some dispute.

The hypothesis is that sexual orientation differences are to some degree the result of genetic or prenatal environmental origins.[44] Homoerotic individuals may fail to follow the normative canalization of one's sex, which suggests that they should by definition be biologically different from heterosexuals of their sex. Often ignored in this formulation is the extent to which gay and straight people share more similarities than differences in their biological makeup. In addition, few acknowledge that the sexuality of same-sex-attracted individuals is different from that of heterosexuals more often in degree than in kind.

Although few researchers propose that all homoerotic individuals vary to the same extent in their deviation from the typical biology of their sex, from a strictly biological perspective, something had to "happen" to create a nonheterosexual individual. This something should be manifested in distinctive, sex-atypical anatomical, neurological, and hormonal variations that inimitably shape an adolescent's physical presentation, perceptions, cognitions, emotions, temperament, behavior, abilities, and even career interests. For example, a body of empirical literature suggests that homosexual individuals differ from heterosexuals in size of certain nuclei in the hypothalamus, in hormonal levels during critical periods of prenatal life when particular sex-related traits are laid down, and in physical features such as shoulder-to-hip ratios, finger length ratio, fingerprint patterns, handedness, and acoustic abilities.[45]

A biological portrayal of homoerotic sexuality presents it as fundamentally sexual inversion. That is, in some respects, gay boys are really heterosexual girls with a penis; and in some respects, lesbian girls are really heterosexual boys without a penis. Sometimes this is carried too far. For example, one characteristic linked with biological sex is age of reaching puberty. Following the sexual inversion model, gay boys should have an early onset of pubescence, because females begin puberty several years before boys; and lesbian girls should have a delayed pubescence, reflecting the later onset of males. One study found that, indeed, gay and bisexual males experience the onset of puberty six months earlier than heterosexual males. This was hypothesized to be the result of differences in the "relevant structures in the nervous system (e.g., sites in the anterior hypothalamus)" between gay and heterosexual males. A similar finding was not confirmed for females, and recently the male data were disconfirmed.[46]

The age-of-pubescence example highlights the tendency for biological research to focus on unique features of nonheterosexuality. The argument is not that every same-sex-attracted boy has an early, sex-atypical pubertal onset, but that sexual orientation differences are apparent at the population level. That is, one cannot predict that a particular boy has same-sex attractions by simply assessing his age of pubertal onset. The "anomaly" of adolescent girls, who actually trend against biological prediction by reporting a slightly *earlier* age of puberty relative to heterosexual girls, remains unexplained, except for the generic and relatively meaningless rationale that different processes affect sexual orientation in women than men.

A second factor proposed as being different for heterosexuals and homosexuals is the impact of socialization. Growing up amidst family members, close friends, schools, religious organizations, and courtrooms that presume and prescribe exclusive heterosexuality is said to influence adolescent development. The effect is believed to be true not only for those with overt same-sex desires and who claim a gay, lesbian, or bisexual identity but also for those who are only subconsciously aware of their same-sex sexuality.

Cultural consequences of sexual orientation differences are difficult for researchers to assess but are nevertheless considered inevitable because of their intuitive appeal. Although adolescents of all sexualities want to feel connected and supported, what might well be unique for same-sex-attracted teens is the effort required and the difficulty inherent in finding others with a shared same-sex orientation. Research suggests that gay-identified youth have smaller social networks, worry more about losing friendships because of their sexuality, believe that fewer romantic relationships are available to them, experience a greater likelihood of compromised relationships with parents, and rate their school's climate and acceptance more negatively.[47] When subjected in schools to the derogatory slur "You're so gay," same-sex-attracted teens are more likely to be affected because they know that indeed they *are* "so gay," as opposed to straight students, who know the slurs are false.

Tony D'Augelli has devoted much of his scholarly career to documenting the ways in which cultural negativity, especially in the form of verbal and physical harassment and violence, shapes gay youth.[48] He argues that victimization leads already vulnerable teens to feel more depressed, more alone, and more suicidal. Even subtle, unspoken messages about the unacceptability of homosexuality may have a negative effect, especially during the vulnerable years of childhood and adolescence. Being rejected by the Boy Scouts or by school jocks or cheerleaders causes teens to lose potential sources of support, comfort, and social interaction that are more easily available to their heterosexual peers.

I am not claiming that all same-sex-attracted teens react identically or even negatively to the cultural reality of gender and sexual expression. Neither am I blind to the fact that some heterosexual young people face similarly difficult challenges when they are tomboys or sissies or they choose not to follow traditional heterosexual scripts but desire, for example, to remain single and focus on their career. I do believe, however, that these negotiations are both more inevitable and more difficult for some same-sex-attracted teens. Dilemmas may well permeate their daily lives in ways not encountered by heterosexual adolescents, who can freely express their sexuality with a lack of deliberation or justification and without fear of scrutiny or evaluation.

NOT MONOLITHIC

The presumption of the first two tenets of both sameness and difference between same- and opposite-sex-attracted adolescents too easily masks the incredible amount of variation *within* each population. Exploring these variations is the most promising area of research on sexual minorities.

The ways in which same-sex-oriented teens vary among themselves may or may not mirror divisions observed in the developmental histories of heterosexuals. The number of characteristics shared by a given subpopulation is boundless. These include both macro factors, such as gender, ethnicity, cohort, and class; and micro factors, such as physical skills, personality characteristics, and real-world experiences. In many cases, these characteristics are so common to a given group as to make any differences across sexual orientations trivial. That is, same-sex-attracted teens, when considering relevant personal characteristics and their status as members of a definable group, may be more similar to heterosexual peers than they are to other gay people.

The possibilities for divergent pathways are endless. A few examples should suffice. The average adolescent girl generally achieves higher levels of intimacy, sensitivity, and empathy in her close relationships than does the average adolescent boy, regardless of sexual orientation. Perhaps as a result, more of the romantic relationships of same-sex-attracted girls than boys evolve from friendships and are characterized by emotional intimacy.[49] A same-sex-attracted boy is more similar to other boys than to lesbians in preferring lustful or novelty sex rather than romantic sex. That is, gender trumps sexual orientation.

As noted earlier, among various ethnic groups, Asian Americans are least likely to disclose their same-sex sexuality to parents and to engage in early same-sex activity and dating.[50] In these matters they are more similar to heterosexual Asian Americans in their understanding of shame and family expectations than they are to non–Asian American gay teens. So, too, same-sex-attracted African American young people have much in common with heteroerotic African Americans. Both must navigate their ethnic identity within white culture, which likely preempts commonalities they share with white gay teens. Or being a member of a double minority may overshadow being either gay or black. Along these lines, if an individual is gay, black, and female, then she is a member of a triple minority with a distinct pathway. If she's also disabled, it's a quadruple minority; if economically disadvantaged, a quintuple minority. Distinct pathways are both common and likely significant.

Sex and ethnic differences are also apparent in school settings. Sexual-minority boys rated their school climate more negatively than did girls, perhaps because of the greater sex-role-conformity demands and sexual orientation victimization experienced by boys. Given their greater need, not surprisingly boys were more positively affected than girls by attending meetings of school-based Gay-Straight Alliances.[51] Hispanic, black, and Asian same-sex-attracted students had fewer negative educational attitudes, experiences, and expectations than white gay teens because, according to one study, at least, young people of color have developed resiliency to prejudice because of their experiences and the support they receive from families.[52]

It is relatively easy to provide these sex and ethnic contrasts. Distinguishing developmental trajectories based on microlevel features is more difficult. The only one that has received much attention is the presence of sex-atypical characteristics. Some same-sex-attracted teens easily pass as straight (and they may "pass" internally as well). Others couldn't do so even if they wanted to. One lesbian adolescent has wide shoulders and narrow hips; while another has a more traditionally feminine body build. Both have a lesbian orientation, but each has a distinctive presentation, and this may affect their life experiences. We don't know. We also don't know the answers to the following questions:

Does playing quarterback on a high school football team imply that a same-sex-attracted athlete identifies more with other athletes than with gay boys?

Do girls who recall adolescent, but not childhood, same-sex desires differ in important ways from those who had sex with other girls during third-grade sleepovers?

Is the boy who has sex before he identifies as gay fundamentally different and therefore destined toward a different future from the boy who knows he's gay without the benefit of best-friend sex?

What distinguishes the girl who has sex with other girls and remains heterosexually identified from the girl who has the same sexual experience and identifies as lesbian?

What distinguishes a boy who eschews a sexual identity label altogether from the boy who identifies himself as gay, comes out, and then "converts" to heterosexuality?

Is a sex-atypical lesbian more intensely same-sex oriented than a sex-typical lesbian in the intensity of her sexual desires, libido, and behavior?[53]

Trying to get into this level of analysis may not be helpful at this point. So little is known about nearly every aspect of same-sex sexuality that to mull over such specific questions feels disingenuous. Even for gender, the within-group comparison receiving the most attention, little is understood about why being a gay female or male seems to matter so much. Perhaps girls will be girls and boys will be boys regardless of sexuality. Or are the cultural stereotypes true—that gay boys are femme and gay girls are butch? Are gay men and lesbians really the other sex, does each of these two groups act like the other sex, and is this a valid way of studying them?

The chapters that follow explore variations between the sexes among same-sex-attracted teenagers. Perhaps sex categorization is valid; or perhaps we tend toward such a sex-difference categorization because of what researchers have chosen to study in the past.

5

Feeling Different

Researchers have learned some things about the genetics and prenatal life of same-sex-attracted individuals.[1] Thus far, however, we have only limited knowledge regarding the genesis of same-sex attractions, arousal, and behavior. It is difficult, at best, to accurately predict future sexuality on the basis of genetics or prenatal environment. The childhood of same-sex-attracted individuals has also been ignored, although some scholars believe that childhood behavior might be a clue to adult homosexuality. The obscurity of the "latency development of prehomosexuals" is almost absolute.[2]

Two points are noteworthy. First, what little is known has been derived from the recalled childhood of adults who currently identify as gay. This is problematic because such accounts can easily be distorted by decades of intervening events and because even if the recollections are accurate, growing up today with same-sex attractions might be very different from the way it was even ten years ago. Second, as can be imagined, childhood narratives of same-sex attractions and behavior are potentially politically explosive because some might believe that such efforts are motivated by the attempt to identify "pregay" children and steer them away from their homosexuality.

Perhaps the best early *subjective* predictor of a same-sex orientation is a child's feeling of being different from peers. *Objectively*, this is usually linked to atypical gender expression. In other words, if "inverted" in one, then "inverted" in the other. Children do not necessarily understand this equation, but adolescents or young adults do. Influenced by the stereotypes of their culture, adolescents with same-sex attractions come to understand that their pervasive sense that something "is not quite right" and their acting like a tomboy or a sissy are the first signs of homosexuality. The implicit assumption here is that all same-sex-oriented teens were indeed sex-atypical children and that all sex-atypical children grow up to be gay. According to researcher Michael Bailey, the second is certainly more true than the first.[3]

In fact, however, little is known about these first manifestations of homoeroticism, other than the average age at which they appear. Their content, meaning, and significance remain mysterious. In the process of recreating the childhood of same-sex-oriented individuals, feelings of differentness and sex atypicality are the usual suspects to be addressed.

First Signs

If gay and straight people differ as adults, then they must also be different as children. We suspect that this is true, but without really knowing why or how this should be. After all, if gay adults had the same kind of childhood as straight adults, how could we tell the difference between the two? How did they become gay? Why are they gay and not straight? Something had to go "wrong" or, more precisely, go differently. Perhaps a certain experience or set of experiences during childhood swayed gay people away from the customary route to heterosexuality. Potential hypotheses—a traumatic experience, bad parenting, physical abuse, early sexual experiences, bad luck—have been more theoretically than empirically driven.

Regardless of what the motivating set of forces may have been, the individual child must have felt this difference, though he or she was unable to verbalize it at the time or identify what the feelings were exactly. Investigators try to determine these things by asking articulate adolescents the leading question "Did you feel different growing up?" A rarely asked question, but one that should be asked, is "How did you feel different?"

If an adolescent girl isn't sure of her sexual attractions, wonders if she might be falling in love with another girl, can't figure out what her sexual identity is, or has an unexplained interest in women who love women, will she feel dissimilar from her peers? If an adolescent boy believes that his homoerotic sexuality is caused by family inheritance, by a prenatal surge of one hormone or another, by bad parenting, by being called "fag" and "sissy," by the drinking water, or by a combination of these hypothetical factors, will he feel dissimilar from his peers? These two young people most likely will believe that their preadolescent life experiences were different from those around them. But don't most adolescents feel this way? Don't most of them think, "No one before me has ever lived my life"?

Setting aside questions of whether, how often, and how much an adolescent feels different during childhood allows one to consider the substantial data and anecdotal reports of how being attracted to someone of the same sex creates a sense of apartness. One review of the literature suggests that feeling different is rooted in childhood experiences of departing from peer norms in concrete ways.[4] Compared to heterosexual boys, gay boys report that they are less aggressive, less conventionally masculine, more overtly feminine, and more inclined toward artistic or scientific endeavors than toward sports, and they feel more erotic interest in other boys. Scholars assume that the opposite pattern holds for lesbian girls who feel out of sync. These characteristics the child supposedly experiences as not a good difference but as a *bad* difference, leading her or him to feel misunderstood, isolated, shamed, suppressed, and internally repressed.

Often not considered are many individuals who cover a range of sexualities—same-sex-oriented individuals who do not identify as gay; who love *both* women and men; who are lesbians who look and act feminine; who are gay males who look and act masculine; who are heterosexuals whose sex-role behavior falls outside the normative range for people of their sex; who are transgender; who do not fit any sexual or sexual orientation scheme but who are nevertheless part of the spectrum of adolescent sexuality.

These complications raise havoc for the sexual identity models discussed in the last chapter. The hallmark of the initial rung of development is the "pregay" child who feels different growing up. For model proposer Richard Troiden, these feelings characterize the "sensitization" stage. At this stage, a child intuits apartness from conventionality but is only dimly (if at all) aware that these feelings have relevance for his or her sexuality.[5]

An early San Francisco study compared the incidence of feeling different among sexual identity groupings.[6] The question asked was: "In grade school, to what extent did you think that you were different from others your age?" About one in five of all respondents, gay and straight alike, reported that they felt "not at all" different from their grade-school peers. Of the 80 percent who did feel varying degrees of differentness, three times as many gay as heterosexual adults felt "very much" different as children. The reasons the gay respondents gave for these feelings were considerably different from the reasons heterosexual respondents gave. The primary, but not sole, reason gay respondents gave had to do with their gender-related traits. Lesbians recalled that their interest in sports made them feel different from other girls. Nearly half of gay men mentioned their *lack* of interest in sports. However, nearly one quarter of heterosexual men also felt different because they were not into sports.

A second reason for feeling different among lesbians and gay men, reported by one in five, was their sexual interest in those of their own gender and their lack of sexual interest in the other gender. Only one in fifty heterosexuals cited this reason. Heterosexual women were the only group that frequently mentioned physical appearance or physical characteristics as a reason for feeling different.

In his sexual identity model, Richard Troiden proposed that the gay person's initial sense of being marginalized is understood in gender terms—not acting or feeling like a typical girl or boy.[7] Children are aware of how a member of their sex is supposed to act at an earlier age than they are aware of what it means to be gay or straight. Nearly half of Troiden's adult gay male respondents attributed their childhood feelings of differentness to gender inadequacies, effeminacy, and lack of masculine interests. They also frequently reported feeling alienated and experiencing a warmth and excitement in the presence of other males. Feeling sexually attracted to the "wrong" sex, which seemed natural to these gay respondents, was considerably less important a source of differentness than feeling gender inappropriateness. By their teenage years, however, 99 percent of the men felt *sexually* different. Strong sexual interest in other boys, waning or nonexistent sexual interest in girls, sexual contact with boys, and feelings of gender inadequacy were the reasons they gave for feeling sexually different. In another study, three quarters of adult lesbians felt different, but only half believed this difference was related to their lesbian identity.[8] Other studies conducted during the same time period with individuals coming of age in the 1950s and 1960s reported similar results.[9]

In recent years, same-sex desires have increasingly appeared in our culture, in forms that touch the lives of young children. During the last decade, therefore, we might expect the age at which young people realize that gendered behavior and sexual orientation are associated to have decreased. Children on grade-school playgrounds have learned to call the sissy boy "fag" and the butch girl "dyke." Some argue that these names have little to do with sexuality per se and more to do with undesirability generally.

It also bears emphasizing that some gay-identified individuals feel

"normal" growing up, have opposite-sex sexual interests, and participate in sex-typical sports, hobbies, and games. In addition, some
straight-identified individuals feel "abnormal" growing up, have
same-sex sexual interests, and participate in sex-atypical sports, hobbies, and games. These are the kinds of individuals who are inad-
vertently overlooked when the connection between adult same-sex
orientation and sex atypicality is drawn.

Another caveat is that most of what we know about feeling different is derived from studies of previous generations of adults, who
were recalling memories of events that occurred decades earlier.
More recent studies tend not to ask participants about childhood
feelings. I am not sure why this is so; perhaps the link between feeling different and having same-sex attractions seems so obvious that
no one thinks it needs further empirical verification.

One recent longitudinal investigation of same-sex-attracted youth
has, however, explored these questions. It found that three quarters of
the boys and two thirds of the girls felt different as children, initially
at the average age of eight years.[10] Somewhat fewer recalled being
called sissy (55 percent) or tomboy (64 percent). Whether these labels and feelings of differentness were linked in the minds of the respondents or the name-callers at the time is not clear. Just over half
recalled being told by someone that they *were* different, and about
one third said their parents tried to stop them from acting like a sissy
or tomboy. Both of these occurred, on average, around ten or eleven
years of age.

As far as I can tell from the limited research, gay adults are slightly
more likely than straight adults to recall feeling different while growing up. In addition, they felt *more* different than straight adults felt,
and they believed that these feelings had (unknown) repercussions
for their future. Although many same-sex-attracted teens feel out of
sync with peers for the same reasons as all adolescents—because of
their looks, their abilities, and their skills—they also carry the potential social burden of their sex-atypical behavioral characteristics. This

burden might be more difficult for boys than for girls because of the social ostracism associated with boyhood femininity. These characteristics are not exclusive to gay young people, but they do appear to be less sex typical than straight youth. Gay boys being less masculine and gay girls being less feminine than their peers (which seems to be more common than gay boys being called sissies and gay girls tomboys) can be problematic. Having erotic fascinations for members of their own sex doesn't seem to bother them so much. These attractions feel natural.

It is the gay person's lack of harmony between biological sex and presentation of self—in other words, sex atypicality—that has been most widely studied. Relatively ignored has been the decreased level of sex typicality generally (boys being less masculine and girls less feminine than heterosexual youth).

Sex Atypicality

The writings of early sexologists Karl Heinrich Ulrichs, Magnus Hirschfeld, Havelock Ellis, Sigmund Freud, and Richard van Krafft-Ebing in the late nineteenth and early twentieth centuries forged the link between homosexuality and gender inversion.[11] In the 1860s Ulrichs maintained that a homosexual male encompassed the soul of a female within an anatomically correct male body. According to Krafft-Ebing, a homosexual woman's body build resembled a man's more than a woman's, with its corresponding masculine frame, pelvis, voice, gait, and penis (enlarged clitoris). Ellis and Freud proposed that all individuals have both masculine and feminine characteristics, and that what distinguishes homosexual from heterosexual individuals is the degree to which sex-atypical features are latent (heterosexual) or overt (homosexual).

Considerable anecdotal evidence suggests that this connection between gender and sexual inversion is not new. Many cultures throughout history have conceived of homosexuality in this way. In detailing the history of gay New York at the turn of the twentieth century, historian George Chauncey defined the terminology used at the time to describe three types of homosexual men:[12]

"Pansy": a man who affected an effeminate manner.
"Queer": a man who looked normal but was attracted to other men.
"Normal": a man interested in women but who would on occasion be the inserter with other men.

Chauncey's evidence suggests that the inversion association exists in many cultural settings and time periods, but is interpreted differently in different cultures and times.

Perhaps more important is the question of how various cultures treat individuals who evince sex-atypicality. "Poorly" is the norm in many Western cultures, at least in regard to effeminacy among males. But not all cultures treat such atypical girls and boys in the same way. In his ethnography of Native American Indians, for example, anthropologist Walter Williams provides examples of "two-spirit" children who nearly all "end up being homosexual," but who are not made to feel the shame instilled in comparable children in Western culture. Williams notes that

American Indian religions view androgynous persons . . . as evidence that that person has been blessed with two spirits. Because both the masculine and the feminine are respected, a person who combines them is considered as higher than the average person, who only has one spirit. Therefore, persons who act like the other sex are not condemned as "deviant" but are blessed for their possession of a double dose of spirituality. They are not "abnormal" but "exceptional."[13]

Given the prevalence of the relationship, a biological connection between an atypical sexual orientation and an atypical gender expression has been made. Thus, the more sex atypical in gender expression, the more "incurable" (congenital) is the homosexual condition assumed to be. Homosexuality is a biological anomaly that is manifested both physically and psychologically. Indeed, this association has been the prevailing working hypothesis of biological research over several decades. The same hormonal or genetic factors that alter the brain to create biologically atypical sexual attractions are believed to be also responsible for fashioning sex-inappropriate behavior, perceptions, cognitions, temperament, and interests.[14]

In reviewing the evidence, social psychologist Anne Peplau suggests that the link might be true of male homosexuality but that the evidence is sparse among women. She warns that "efforts to present universal theories of sexual orientation that apply to both sexes have tended to take male experiences as the norm, much to the detriment of our understanding of women."[15]

SCIENTIFIC EVIDENCE FOR THE INVERSION ASSOCIATION

Few are so naïve as to suggest that the correlation between sexual and gender inversion is perfect. However, so convinced were early researchers about the intimate link between effeminacy and homosexuality that they refused to believe that masculine gay boys existed. In his review of the Terman-Miles study, the first empirical investigation of sexual orientation and gender, Theo Sandfort points out that the homosexual male sample was divided by the investigators into the active and the passive. "Active" homosexuals were those who preferred the inserter role in sexual activity with other men; these "masculine" men were dropped from further consideration in the study. No explanation for this decision was deemed necessary. Vestiges of this division into "true" and "false" homosexuals can be observed in some Latin cultures, although this is less so as the Westernized, *modernos* gay man has emerged.[16] He may be both inserter and insertee.

Since the Terman-Miles study, investigators have relied less frequently on specific roles assumed during sex acts, perhaps because most gays and lesbians are versatile, like most human beings, when it comes to sex positions. Rather, personality traits, behaviors, and interests that have a known sex bias have become the measures of choice. Sometimes femininity and masculinity are conceptualized as resting on opposite poles of a single psychological continuum. The more a girl is feminine, the less she can be masculine. Others emphasize a multidimensional approach. Individuals can score high or low on femininity and high or low on masculinity. Four "types" are thus possible: feminine (high femininity/low masculinity), masculine (low femininity/high masculinity), androgynous (high femininity/ high masculinity), and undifferentiated (low femininity/low masculinity).[17]

Several early studies drew the connection between femininity or masculinity and sexual orientation in children and adolescents. Usually, they included boys who had been referred to the researchers by parents because of concern with their son's girl-like qualities. Richard Green's *The Sissyboy Syndrome* is the classic study of this type.[18] The boys felt soft, liked to cuddle with their mothers, played with dolls, dressed up as girls, abhorred the violence and aggressiveness of male games, befriended girls and not boys, and expressed a desire to be a girl. In a few cases, they wanted their penis removed. Their girl-like behavior extended to their erotic desires and sexual behavior. As they became adolescents and young adults, nearly all of these extremely sissy boys reported sexual attraction to other males.[19]

Green's sissy boys are extreme cases. More commonly, researchers ask a range of adults to recall their child and adolescent play behavior and interests. One study questioned nearly 800 adults living in the Los Angeles area about such activities.[20] Although gay adults were more likely than heterosexuals to remember sex-atypical interests, the children did not vary in their enjoyment of common activities, including climbing, hide-and-seek, reading, bicycling, and going to the movies. These activities were independent of the respondents' sexual orientation or sex.

It bears emphasizing that many activities and interests, especially during childhood, are not sex typed. Equally important, sex-linked characteristics are not absolute. Some might be sex linked at one time or in one culture (girls playing team sports; boys wearing a necklace) but not in others. A third potential source of error is to assume that the sexes are equally likely to have their sexual orientation and sex atypicality linked.

SEX ATYPICALITY AMONG GIRLS

Given the prevailing notion of inversion, if a girl desires girls (a masculine trait), then she must also mimic boys in other ways. She would be likely to be interested in, for example, racing cars, fighting, building forts, playing with balls, climbing trees, hunting, and reading adventure books. She would not be interested in dressing up dolls, dancing, jumping rope, playing house, skipping, cooking, and reading romance books. She would dress like a boy, hate skirts and long hair, and want to be a boy and not a girl. She would aspire to traditionally male jobs—doctor, lawyer, engineer; she would not want to be a nurse, legal secretary, or receptionist. She would be aggressive, cavalier, courageous, and ambitious, not emotional, affectionate, talkative, and patient. She would avoid children, cosmetics, and long-term relationships. She'd be a hunter, not a gatherer. She'd be a tomboy—a butch, not a femme—from an early age.

This picture, however, does not match what we know about same- versus opposite-sex-attracted girls. Few girls have such extreme gender dysphoria as Green's sissy boys seem to have. And those few who do show these characteristics do not necessarily become lesbians. A longitudinal study of young women found that recalled childhood and adolescent sex atypicality failed to predict sexual questioning or eventual sexual identity.[21] One review of the research suggested that the association between the two is, at best, weak: "The links among masculinity, femininity, and women's sexual orientation are variable rather than constant across cultures and historical periods. Far from holding the key to understanding women's sexual orientation, the adoption of masculine or feminine characteristics may reflect prevailing cultural norms and values."[22] The one study usually cited as the evidence for sexual orientation differences among women actually demonstrates mixed results.[23] Even though the lesbian participants in the study lived in San Francisco, attended lesbian-oriented social and political events, and went to women-only bars in the 1960s, differences between them and heterosexual women in gender-related behavior were not as great as they were for men. True, compared to the straight women, the lesbian-identified women seldom recalled participating in typical girl activities. But only slightly more than half of heterosexual women recalled these activities. True, the lesbians in the study more often recalled preferring the activities of boys, wearing boys' clothes, and pretending to be a boy. But only one third of the lesbians reported extreme versions of masculine behavior. For activities deemed neither masculine nor feminine, no sexual orientation differences were found. On childhood personality characteristics, sexual orientation effects were even sparser. Lesbians were more likely to recall being dominant and independent children compared to the heterosexual women.

In examining these patterns, it is essential to keep in mind a critical fact: psychological gender is different from behavioral gender. A girl can "walk like a man" (behavioral) but be sensitive and emotional (psychological). With that distinction in mind, consider the following points gleaned from an analysis of the existing literature on sex atypicality and homosexuality in women:[24]

Lesbian and heterosexual women do not differ on psychological femininity or androgyny.

Lesbians rate themselves modestly higher on psychological masculinity measures, although this may be due to sampling biases (recruiting feminist-oriented lesbians).

Masculine characteristics lesbians are more likely to assign to themselves include independence, a willingness to take risks, a strong personality, self-sufficiency, and decisiveness.

Behavioral deviations from one's biological sex are somewhat better predictors of women's sexual orientation than psychological deviations; in the case of women, these behavioral differences are frequently subsumed under the rubric "tomboy." Adult lesbians recall higher levels of childhood gender nonconformity than heterosexual women do. The strongest predictors of female homosexuality are cross-dressing and having a reputation as a tomboy. However, the link between even tomboyishness and sexual orientation is weak.[25] Of the many gender-related activities and personality characteristics that have been assessed, relatively few can identify homoerotic, as opposed to heteroerotic, girls.

Why is this the case? The usual explanation is that the cultural stigma attached to girls playing boy-type games is considerably less that it is for boys playing girl-type games. Few straight boys dare be caught playing house, hopscotch, or jacks, even if they really liked these games. Girls playing aggressive sports, associating with boys, and wanting to be mechanics, airline pilots, and soldiers are more common and more apt to be rewarded. Parents are seldom upset when their daughter manifests male-typical behavior, probably because it suggests experimentation, power, and prestige in a way that girly behavior rarely can among boys. In one study, 77 percent of lesbians and 63 percent of heterosexual women reported being tomboys while growing up.[26] This finding suggests that the overwhelming majority of tomboys will grow up to be straight women.[27]

Michael Bailey's Tomboy Project, a longitudinal study of four- to nine-year-old girls identified by their parents as tomboys, will eventually provide critical answers to many of these long-standing and perplexing issues.[28] The study probes its subjects' developmental histories, including the nature of the girls' sexual and romantic lives. At the initial interview, although tomboys proved to be more similar to their brothers than to their sisters in toy and activity preferences, they were less masculine than their brothers. Bailey plans to assess whether the tomboys as adolescents will be attracted to girls or boys, have sex with girls or boys, and desire to date girls or boys.

The connection between sexual orientation and sex-atypical psychological and behavioral expression has been both more frequently explored and confirmed among boys than girls. Even here, however, we must provide a caveat. The link is stronger in matters regarding boys' deficiencies in masculinity rather than their overt expressions of femininity.

SEX ATYPICALITY AMONG BOYS

The logic for the association between gender and sexual inversion in boys is similar to that for girls. If a boy desires boys—considered a feminine trait—then he is a sissy and would have other female characteristics. He would, for example, despise football, baseball, fighting, and hunting. He occupies the artistic and creative realms, which are considered to be feminine. One consequence of these boys' femininity is that they receive considerable ridicule from peers, which peaks during late childhood and junior high school and declines during the course of high school. "Gayson," "Wimp," "Tinkerbell," "Pansy," and "Avon Lady" are among the notable epithets.[29]

The San Francisco study, data for which was gathered nearly forty years ago, is frequently cited to support the association between same-sex attraction in males and feminization.[30] As adults, the men in the study rarely recalled engaging in typical masculine activities as children and adolescents. Only one in ten gay men, compared to seven in ten heterosexual men, played baseball and football. Few described themselves as very strong or active as children. Although nearly half took pleasure in stereotypical girls' activities, such as playing house, hopscotch, and jacks, the respondents' primary preference was for solitary games and activities not associated with gender, such as drawing, music, and reading. Summarizing their childhood play preferences, the gay male adults recalled being somewhat more feminine, clearly more gender neutral, and decidedly less masculine than was suggested by the memories recalled by heterosexual men. Furthermore, memories of childhood gender nonconformity were the strongest predictors of adult gay men experiencing same-sex arousal, sex with other males, and a gay identity.

Although sexual orientation differences in childhood play activities are often quite marked, it bears noting that these are memories, not observations, of behavior. Furthermore, not all gay-identified men fit either a childhood sissy-boy syndrome or an attenuated version of it—the absence of both masculinity and femininity. Consider the following data about gay men, also from the San Francisco study:

There were no sexual orientation differences between gay and straight men in their feelings of dominance and independence.

One quarter of gay men felt not very weak but very strong as children.

Nearly half recalled having a very active boyhood.

Nearly one in five reported being very masculine.

Over half did not enjoy sissy-type games; 10 percent of heterosexual men did.

Most had never dressed in girls' clothes or pretended to be girls.

Other data confirm these observations.[31] Notably, it is the absence of childhood masculine traits rather than the presence of feminine traits that is the better predictor of a same-sex orientation.[32] In the Los Angeles study, homosexual boys were similar to heterosexual girls in their low level of participation in team sports but similar to heterosexual boys in their low level of engagement in girl-typical activities.[33] Thus, scientifically speaking, what distinguishes straight from gay men is more the absence of masculine traits than the existence of feminine ones. It's not that gay boys are such sissies but that they're not such great butches.

Table 5.1   Scores in play activities

Sex by orientation grouping	Feminine score	Masculine score
Heterosexual girls	17.6	7.5
Homosexual girls	11.8	11.3
Heterosexual boys	6.2	12.9
Homosexual boys	10.0	8.3

Source: Grellert, Newcomb, & Bentler, 1982.

GIRLS AND BOYS, GAYS AND STRAIGHTS

When it comes to recalled memories of liking team sports and rough-and-tumble play, heterosexual boys score highest, followed by same-sex-attracted girls, same-sex-attracted boys, and, finally, heterosexual girls. On playing with dolls, playing house, and playing the piano, heterosexual girls score highest, followed by same-sex-attracted boys and girls, and heterosexual boys. One study's feminine/ masculine scores in play activities are presented in Table 5.1 to illustrate these trends (no ranges are given in the original).[34]

Based solely on reports of play activities, researchers claim that they can correctly assign 70 percent to 90 percent of all adults into their appropriate sexual orientation grouping.[35] Because femininity scores are usually more broadly distributed than masculine scores, they serve as better predictors. Hence, heterosexual boys are said to be the easiest to predict because of their extreme aversion to feminine behavior and their strong preference for boys' games. At the other end of the spectrum, same-sex-attracted girls are the most diverse and thus the most difficult to place in the correct group.[36] In general, heterosexual children (especially boys) appear more invested than same-sex-attracted boys and girls in "culturally appropriate" sex-typed behavior.

It is critical to remember that these predictions based on childhood play behavior are far from perfect. In addition, these predictions are usually derived from the reports of self-identified gay and lesbian adults, not the much larger population of nonidentified or undisclosed individuals with same-sex desires. Further complicating these reservations, the overlap among sexual orientation groupings is even more pronounced when the two categories are expanded to three, to include bisexuals. Whether bisexually oriented individuals are at the midpoint in their gender expression or more similar to gays or straights is hotly contested. The limited evidence suggests that bisexuals of both sexes are more diverse and thus more often "misclassified" than either heterosexuals or lesbians and gay men based on their childhood play associations and behavior.[37] Intriguing data presented by Kenneth Cohen provide a partial solution to this dilemma. Cohen separated masculinity from femininity scores. He found that bisexual college men were midway between gay and heterosexual men in masculinity scores, but were more similar to gay men than heterosexual men in their level of femininity.[38] Similar data are needed for women.

Another polarizing issue based on sexual orientation differences in sex atypicality is contained in Daryl Bem's "exotic becomes erotic" (EBE) theory. Bem asserts that biological differences among children prompt some to engage in more female-typical play activities and others in male-typical ones.[39] Usually these preferences are consistent with one's biological sex, but not always. Children whose play is not consistent with their biological sex become "pregays," according to Bem. Critics of EBE theory have focused primarily on its lack of applicability to the lives of women.[40]

The data presented in this chapter show little support for the unique sex atypicality of girls who will eventually identify as lesbian. If we knew the full scope of same-sex attractions among boys, I believe the same would hold true for them. The young men and women I interviewed did not provide support for EBE theory. Few of the young lesbians as girls were classically butch or masculine in their friendships and play activities, and only a minority of gay males fit the classic sissy stereotype.

First, consider the girls. Only one in three engaged in team and individual sports and had primarily boys as friends. Only several as children were teased about being lesbian or masculine. One in two reported that they were not into stereotypically boy activities, or reported that they had any male friends. They much preferred girls as friends. At most, perhaps one third of the girls is a candidate to support EBE theory. Clearly, one half is not.

The same-sex-attracted boys conformed slightly better to EBE theory. One in two preferred girls as friends. They were on average teased daily or weekly because of their gender expression or, less frequently, their sexual orientation. In addition, the majority disliked typically male activities and sports. Inconsistent with EBE theory, however, these boys did not turn to typically female activities for enjoyment, and fully one in four had exclusively boys as friends. At best, perhaps one half of the boys is a candidate to support EBE theory. Clearly, one quarter is not.

The majority of young adults I spoke with did not see themselves as either butch or femme. This has proven to be a particularly difficult pill for those who ascribe to some form of a gender or sexual inversion theory. Many are quick to ignore the overwhelming diversity of gender expression among same-sex-oriented children and adolescents. Within-group variability for each sexual orientation grouping is so pronounced as to dwarf any other consideration.[41] A differential developmental trajectories perspective acknowledges such diversity.

Feeling Different and Gender Expression

Surprisingly little is known about the childhood of same-sex-oriented individuals. What we do know, as we have seen, relies on the recalled memories of adults many years and, at times, decades beyond the actual experience of these feelings and activities. Whether this distance distorts those respondents' memories is unknown, but it should give us pause in making strong statements.

The fact is, childhood feelings of differentness have proven to be at best a poor indicator of future sexual status. Too many homoerotic children did not feel different and too many heteroerotic ones did. Same-sex-oriented individuals are slightly more likely than heterosexual peers to recall having felt different as a child—for some of the same reasons, but to different degrees. Most striking, however, is the degree of diversity among the same-sex-oriented when it comes to such things as whether they felt different, the degree to which they felt different, what the feelings were about, and the impact those feelings had on their future. In these domains researchers need to know a lot more.

Findings regarding sexual orientation differences in gender expression may be partially deceptive. Research design problems may overdetermine the association. First, if sex-atypical same-sex-attracted individuals are more likely to identify and disclose to others that they are gay and do so at earlier ages, they will be more apt to volunteer as research participants and hence are likely to be oversampled. This fact is likely to skew what we know about same-sex-attracted children and adolescents. Second, few studies assess the gender expression of individuals when they are children and adolescents, and it is rare to find confirmation of any report of gender expression by someone other than the subject. One study that did use confirmation by others (in this case, mothers) found reasonable accuracy regarding subjects' reports of childhood sex atypicality.[42]

Yet sissy gay boy and butch gay girl stereotypes thrive. Statistically, on average they are true, at least for those who have participated in the studies. Such stereotypes keep us from seeing the masculine gay male, the feminine lesbian, and the individual who creates a unique blend of gender characteristics. They might also keep us from searching for more telling features that distinguish sexual orientation groupings.

One potential candidate is that, as children, same-sex-attracted boys and girls tend to be loners. This possibility suggested itself to me as I interviewed college students. Many did not feel that they had fit in with their peers. A young man recalled "walking around the city, basically looking at other people . . . creative, imaginative play. Discovering and enjoying spending a lot of time on bike trips, going to new places. Getting out of the house and being outside, just wandering off by myself."[43] A young woman said, "I did math, kept track of things by counting them, built things in the garden, anything analytic. I played a lot alone, running outside a lot."

Other data support these respondents' memories. Gay individuals are more likely to feel alienated during childhood or adolescence.[44] One (traditional) explanation is that same-sex-attracted children are more likely to be rejected by peers and hence become loners because they are different or strange, or evince sex-atypical behavior. Another possibility is that these boys and girls select solitude of their own volition, perhaps because of their creativity, imagination, and intelligence. Investigating this prospect not as a distinctive, defining characteristic of same-sex attraction but as an alternate route to understanding the childhood of such individuals casts a more positive spin on their lives—and is surely a legitimate avenue of inquiry.

Perhaps the most reliable indicator of "gayness" is the emergence of distinctive same-sex attractions. Many scholars consider this to be the first significant milestone in the development of the gay adolescent. This is the subject of the next chapter.

6

Same-Sex Attractions

Our ignorance about the appearance of same-sex attractions and first sexual contact is a subset of the silence regarding the sexuality of prepubertal children—and perhaps also of early adolescents. Perhaps people think that if child sexuality remains unacknowledged, no one will think of children as sexual—or that if children are sexual their sexuality is meaningless and can be ignored. Those who defy or transcend this unspoken accord engender wrath. Ask Judith Levine, author of the provocative book *Harmful to Minors: The Perils of Protecting Children from Sex* (2002). She says that because of long-standing timidity in the United States, "It is nearly impossible to publish a book that says children and teenagers can have sexual pleasure and be safe too." The point of her book—that sexuality can be a "vehicle to self-knowledge, love, healing, creativity, adventure, and intense feelings of aliveness"—is disregarded.[1] Rather, we seem bent on portraying youthful sexuality as treacherous.[2] If we can't talk about childhood heterosexuality generally, imagine the suspicions directed at those who acknowledge or, even worse, advocate for nonnormative sexuality.

Why the reticence?

a. We believe children are asexual, so we are loathe to ask for fear we may find out otherwise.
b. We can't easily identify prepubertal gay children and question them.
c. We believe that gayness arrives with adolescence or the onset of puberty.
d. All of the above.

Answer: d.

A few scholars have managed to resist the pressure to remain silent on this topic. They assert that prepubertal children experience and enjoy sexual feelings, stimulation, and exploration. However, "professional ethics" and cultural norms preclude the systematic collection of this information. If you need verification of this, select any basic professional text on child development and turn to the section that discusses sexual feelings or behavior. You'll find that such a section does not exist, except perhaps under a heading on sexual abuse. Puberty is invariably seen as the starting point for sexual development. But what do we do about children who have sexual attractions and activity prior to puberty? This is the subject of the present chapter and the next.

Emergence

Although sexual desires and attractions are an essential part of adolescent sexuality, scant attention is given to their origin or prevalence during childhood. Except, perhaps, for a nod to boyhood sexuality, the implicit (but incorrect) presumption is that sexual arousal first appears at puberty. Nevertheless, some children—and not all are boys—have frequent and intense sexual desires and fantasies. Whether these have long-term implications for a person's adult sexuality is unknown. Such data are difficult, if not impossible, to collect in the face of the political, financial, and logistical obstacles that hinder developmental research on child sexuality.[3]

In an attempt to avoid the pitfalls of prediction reviewed in the last chapter, investigators pose what they believe to be a more reliable indicator of "gayness"—the emergence of distinctively same-sex attractions. Among the first to study this subject were Alfred Kinsey and his colleagues. They found the median age of first "erotic arousal" in their total sample to be eight years for boys but nearly twice that for girls (age fifteen).[4] Girls were more likely than boys to be erotically aroused by psychological rather than physical stimulation. Thoughts, fantasies, and imagination were central to their eroticism. This is not to say that girls didn't also engage in sexual behavior such as petting and masturbation. Unlike their brothers, however, same-sex sex play was only a minor source of first erotic arousal.

Since Kinsey, interest in the timing of first homosexual and, to a lesser degree, heterosexual attractions among those who identify as gay, lesbian, or bisexual has continued.[5] This overriding interest has been inspired in large part by the desire to document the onset of the first stage of sexual identity development, variously termed "identity confusion," "awareness of attractions," "pre–coming out," "incongruence," and "signification."

Although in all sexual identity models the emergent gay person is supposed to feel somehow out of sorts, different, confused, but erotically connected to others of the same sex, these matters are not investigated. What exactly is the content of the young gay person's eroticism? How do same-sex attractions alter the significance and meaning of early memories for one's life course? Rather, researchers seem to prefer to focus only on the timing of the first signs of an incipient same-sex sexuality.

A first memory of same-sex attractions is not as reliable a marker for same-sex sexuality as you might imagine. Although 80 percent of the same-sex-attracted young men and 60 percent of the young women I interviewed recalled having prepubertal same-sex attractions, the attractions were often not distinct from other developmental milestones, such as first sex or first infatuation. Further complicating matters, some heterosexual young people experience same-sex attractions and some same-sex-attracted young people experience heterosexual attractions.

Researchers know more about the existence of these opposite-sex attractions than they do about the same-sex attractions of heterosexuals. Lesbian girls are usually considered to be more dual-sex oriented than boys. In one study, 100 percent of gay and lesbian adolescents acknowledged same-sex sexual attractions and fantasies, but over 80 percent of the girls and 60 percent of the boys also acknowledged heterosexual attractions, fantasies, and/or arousal.[6] One young woman I interviewed said, "My sophomore year in high school I was sure I was a heterosexual woman because I was mesmerized by boys." Another told me, "I was boy crazy during junior high school and my mom was fine about that, but I just didn't want to date so I never saw the sexual side to it. I just wanted to see if they would like me, and once they did then I didn't like them anymore." Although boys and girls did not substantially differ in age of first same-sex attraction, this was not the case regarding heterosexual attraction. Boys reported heterosexual attraction at the same age as same-sex attraction, a year or two earlier than girls.

It is extraordinarily difficult to locate comparable studies of heterosexual children or adolescents that assess the commencement of their same- or opposite-sex attractions. One existing study reported that among heterosexual women, the average age of first romantic or sexual attraction to males was eleven years.[7] This was the same age as lesbians recalled attractions to females. Two thirds of the heterosexuals and nearly half of the lesbians reported romantic or sexual attractions counter to their sexual orientation—but at differing ages: eighteen years for heterosexuals and thirteen years for lesbians.

Further complicating our understanding of these issues are data from the same study's bisexual women. Nearly all recalled having same-sex attractions, at the average age of thirteen years; somewhat fewer (85 percent) recalled opposite-sex attractions, at a considerably younger average age, ten years. Thus, in the timing of their attractions to males, bisexual women resembled heterosexual women. In the timing of their attractions to females, they more closely paralleled lesbians.[8] Perhaps sexual and romantic attractions consistent with one's sexual orientation emerge during pre- or early puberty and attractions that are inconsistent surface after the onset of puberty. It is worth noting that the information on attraction in this study is incompatible with the traditional view of bisexuality as being either a transitory stage toward lesbianism or toward heterosexuality. The data are compatible, however, with the view that bisexuality is a legitimate sexual orientation.

One final note on this study. By comparing these data to studies on males, the authors concluded that more females than males have cross-orientation attractions. This might well reflect the cultural message received by girls that erotic attractions consist of physical or romantic feelings directed toward boys and that emotional or intimate attractions are directed toward girls.

Timing

Sexual attractions exist among many children and adolescents. When they first become apparent is a source of debate. Researchers' thoughts on the timing of sexual attractions have undergone a dramatic generational change.

THE MAGICAL AGE OF TEN

Conventional wisdom presumes that sexual attractions emerge only after a person's gonadal hormones escalate during the first few years of pubescence. This view has been challenged by researchers Martha

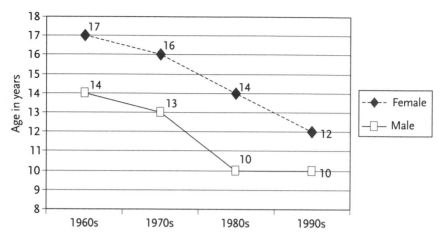

Figure 6.1 Average age of first same-sex attraction

McClintock and Gil Herdt, who argue that sexual attractions are biologically instigated several years prior to the onset of gonadal pubescence, during adrenarche, the time when the adrenal glands mature and produce elevated levels of sex steroids.[9] Sexual feelings may be intensified by pubertal developments, but this is merely an amplification, a ratcheting up of what adrenarche has already made present several years earlier.

Although I basically agree with their analysis, what McClintock and Herdt fail to explain are contrary data regarding the genesis of sexual attractions. Yes, sexuality is energized prior to pubertal onset; but sexual desire, attractions, even behavior are present far in advance of adrenarche for many. Beginning with Kinsey, boys have reported initial erotic imagery prior to adrenarche. Yet as Figure 6.1 illustrates, the average age of first same-sex attractions has only recently reached what has been called the "magical" age of ten, and only for boys. Throughout fifty years of research, the average onset of same-sex arousal has seldom hovered around adrenarche, but occurs years later.

Young women may never remember a time in their life when they were not attracted to other girls. They might not realize at the time, at age three or five or seven, that these feelings toward females have an erotic, sexual content or that they have long-term meaning for how the girls will eventually relate to boys and to other girls. But the feelings are present nevertheless, and they are often a significant and gratifying aspect of their first memories of their young life.

Melissa, for one, could not recall a time in her life when she was not attracted to other girls. When I asked her when she began having same-sex attractions, she responded:

> Forever! And before that! Before school at least. These feelings were always there, and I don't know why, but I guess I was born with them. I don't like dissecting my childhood or figuring out the why of the way I am, but I'll tell you, since you asked.
>
> I've always gotten along better with girls, maybe not the butch girls or the prissy ones who have their noses stuck up, you know, and only aspire to fuck boys. But generally, you know, I liked them, girls, more than boys. I always, always had my girl-friends and felt closer to them. I was always their best friend, the devoted, loyal one, and we did everything together. I can't really recall having a single male friend, unless you count my cousins.[10]

As this example illustrates, it is critical to remember that the average age of ten for first sexual attractions cited in contemporary studies is merely that, the average, with extreme variations from that age reported in nearly every study. Many boys and girls are similar to Melissa: they recall having sexual feelings long before adrenarche kicks in. These memories are often among the first of their lives. But for others, such as Laura, first memories of same-sex attractions emerge long after pubertal onset.

Laura's parents immigrated from the Philippines to Manhattan before she was born. Laura generally ignored dating or a sexual life as she strove through high school to achieve her goal of getting into an

Ivy League university. Then, quite unexpectedly, her life was irrevocably altered. As she recalled:

I was taking this Women Studies course and this TA for the class I couldn't get out of my mind! It wasn't that she was this incredibly beautiful chick or that she was so well dressed, but [there was] just something slick about her. I don't know what to say. I just can't explain it—and I've tried many times. I'm sorry I can't help you more. Like, I'd go to her office hours all the time for the stupidest of things. I was not sure what was going on or what I wanted. And it's not that she helped me that much on my paper, or that I had anything really to ask her, honestly. Nothing ever happened, but I realize now it was a developing crush.[11]

Tony D'Augelli reported that he found that the age of first same-sex awareness among males ranged from prior to two years of age to twenty.[12]

Given this evidence, I am not convinced that adrenarche is the key factor in the emergence of sexual attractions. It may be for some and not others. Same-sex desire may have its genesis in late childhood, but individuals are unwilling to admit it until they feel more comfortable with their homosexuality, which tends to happen only during later adolescence. But how do we account for the very large number of individuals who recall same-sex attractions years before adrenarche? Another question, this one prompted by the McClintock-Herdt findings: Is there a link with adrenarche for heterosexual attractions among same-sex-attracted individuals? And are the opposite- and same-sex attractions of heterosexuals also associated with the magical age of ten?

COHORT CHANGES

Though the specific age of first same-sex attractions is a matter of some debate, there is unmistakable evidence that the average age of recalling first same-sex attractions has dropped precipitously during the past fifty years, from late adolescence to late childhood (as shown in Figure 6.1). Although it is true that questions such as "When did you first realize that you were romantically or sexually attracted to other girls/boys?" were seldom given to those who came of age in the 1950s and 1960s, those who were asked responded that they became aware of same-sex attractions after entering junior high school (boys) or senior high (girls). By the 1980s, age of first awareness had declined to just before junior high school graduation. This age has continued to spiral downward in succeeding years and now averages ten years for boys and twelve years for girls—and may even be younger in urban areas where sexual visibility is at its peak. Whether the average age has stopped declining, whether it is not likely to appreciably decline below the magical age of ten, must await future research.

This steady generational decrease cannot logically be attributed to biology. Age of pubertal onset has not declined so dramatically. It can better be linked with cultural shifts in awareness of same-sex desires and with changes in the questions researchers ask and who are asked them. Although a connection with cultural visibility has not, to the best of my knowledge, been demonstrated, I believe this to obvious. Why a young person might now report her first attractions at age eight and not eighteen is likely related to the increased visibility of alternative sexualities in the media. A name and a meaning have been given to her formerly unspecified and seemingly inconsequential feelings. For example, one Web site tracks the dramatic growth of gay characters on television from the inferred gayness of characters in the 1950s, such as the Cisco Kid and Annie Oakley, to the present array of explicitly gay characters and themes.[13] If modeling affects behavior, there are plenty of models now available to teens. And these models confirm that attractive, athletic, popular, and desirable others can have same-sex attractions. A plurality of images, both real and fictitious, exist with which to match one's persona and desires.

Tara, a high school senior in a Missouri suburb, told me that her sexual attractions to women go "way back. I just don't like the male figure, no offense! My physical attractions are like that, exclusively oriented to the female shape." Tara is "out to the entire world, except my parents." Her Catholic parents are very conservative and have been somewhat suspicious of her friends and her "lifestyle, you know, my women-oriented activities." She recalls:

I was not into He-Man but She-Ra on Saturday morning cartoons. I never missed an episode and oriented my life around her. She-Ra this and She-Ra that. I loved watching her, but I was afraid that friends would notice what I was watching. Maybe I was obsessed with her, but it wasn't just to her. I just loved women![14]

DIFFERENCES BETWEEN BOYS AND GIRLS

In addition to generational changes, it has long been suspected that boys, regardless of sexual orientation, become cognizant of their sexual interests and impulses before girls do. It's not that boys are sexual and girls aren't; it's simply that boys tend to report having sexual attractions at younger ages and tend to describe them differently. Here, sex differences trump sexual orientation differences—that is, heterosexual and gay boys are more alike than gay boys are to lesbians.

The origin of these differences remains open to debate and raises fundamental questions about the relative role of biological and environmental factors. Are there biological (hormonal) differences between girls and boys in the objective strength and intensity of sexual desire? If so, are these as strong as socialization factors that discourage girls from acknowledging or attending to their experiences of sexual arousal but that encourage boys to do so? One uncontested assertion is that female sexuality is more malleable and mutable. That is, female sexuality is more responsive than male sexuality to cultural and social factors, more subject to change in response to external circumstances, and more variable within a particular life course.[15] This is illustrated in the following narrative of a seventeen-year old girl.

I'm more attracted to males, but this is not always true. Attractions to females just take longer to develop. No—that's not true. The time it takes is the same lots of times. Thinking about the attractions is the same—well, I've never counted, but they should be. Right? But it depends, on what I'm not really sure, but it does. In terms of my relationship history, it is easier with males and is more frequent, but then I'm around more males so that's not really fair to the females.

Regardless of the role of biology and socialization, we would be deluding ourselves were we to think that these differences between girls and boys only begin during adolescence. They can be tracked among children of all ages.

Whatever the cause, it needs to be sufficiently strong to account for the dramatic lowering of the age at which girls recall sexual desire. Indeed, both girls and boys can recall being "erotically aroused" at ages that stretch back to first memories of their lives. Or their first arousal can be quite recent. On average, however, boys report prepubertal sexual interests and arousals, which is several years earlier than most girls. The sex difference, however, is lessening. Girls are catching up. When Melissa answers, "Forever! And before that!" to the question of when she first became aware of same-sex attractions, she is reflecting a growing trend. Age of first same-sex awareness is decreasing more rapidly among contemporary adolescent girls than among boys.[16]

MEASUREMENT PROBLEMS

Underlying these age, cohort, and sex differences are legitimate questions about when and how the information is gathered and who is asked to provide it. Most of what we know about first sexual aware-ness is derived by asking a single question requesting age of occur-rence, from gay-identified individuals only. The decreasing age of first attractions might be attributed to the fact that investigators are now asking young adults these questions when the respondents are only a decade or so removed from the actual first occurrence of their same-sex attractions, as well as the fact that such attractions are less taboo now than they were in the 1950s, when they were labeled ille-gal, pathological, and sinful. Recent investigations are studying indi-viduals who are less likely to be retrospectively biased and more likely to recall an early awareness of their sexuality.

In addition, we cannot even be sure that various studies are refer-encing the same thing. One study asked about sexual attractions, fantasies, and arousal to erotica—all factors commonly used by re-searchers as an indication of first same-sex awareness. Yet these three events seldom occurred simultaneously and averaged nearly two years apart[17]—a substantial discrepancy, which suggests that when first sexual arousal occurs is dependent on what question is asked, which has also changed.

Early studies asked about when the respondent "first realized you were gay or somehow different" or was "first aware you were sexually attracted by a male/female." Realization and awareness about being gay are cognitive processes more likely to elicit answers involving later ages than questions that probe emotions and feelings. This real-ization of differentness would probably not emerge until peer com-parisons are possible.

I am also not sure that participants mean what researchers mean by "sexual attraction." Few investigators provide clear definitions of such attraction.[18] Sexual arousal to erotica might not be how some experience their first attractions. Girls and boys may differ. Girls might relate better to questions about sexual fantasies or romantic at-tractions, and boys to physical turn-ons or pornography. A person might have a memory that is singular to that person—for example, a girl's attachment to a best friend that does not apply to anyone else. Maybe she wouldn't have labeled this feeling as being indicative of same-sex attractions at the time she felt it, but she may later recognize that it has meaning beyond the particular friend.

In a case like this, what should count—when the person felt the attachment or when the recognition of its meaning took hold? One young man I interviewed responded to "What age did you first have same-sex attractions?" with his own question: "Do you mean what age did I know they were sexual or what age do I now recognize that I was attracted to other guys?" He was making an important distinction—sexual attractions exist before an understanding of what they mean exists. Without brain imaging or eye dilation data being collected at the time of the experience, it is likely impossible to know with certainty when same-sex attractions first emerge for a particular individual. Our respondents might not even know themselves. Perhaps researchers might edge a little closer to the truth by adding to this question the caveat "You need not have interpreted the attractions as sexual in nature at that time." For example, I ask the following:

Describe your first memories of being attracted to girls/boys. How old were you and what specifically do you remember? You need not have interpreted the attractions as sexual in nature at that time. How far back can you recall such an experience? What did they mean to you at the time? Of what significance did they have? Did they impact other aspects of your life?

Patience on the part of the interviewer can elicit additional information, as the young respondents revise their answers, and as one memory evokes earlier ones. One young woman first denied having any sexual memories from her childhood—except maybe for a time when she was five. "I wanted to move my cot next to the cute girls, and I'd wished I was napping with them as I went to sleep. Being held or holding, touching them. These were my dreams when I woke up from my nap." Then another memory startled her to a further realization. She recalled something from two years earlier, when she was three: "I always wanted to color the pretty girls in coloring books, and I'd color nothing else. I'd just leave the boys in black and white!" Now fully engaged, she excitedly recalled being at her grandmother's house and seeing her uncle's new wife: "I thought she was the most beautiful woman in the world! She had to be a movie star, with such grace and elegance. I just associated the *Flashdance* song 'Let's Get Physical' to her. It was the physical connection to the feelings."[19]

My listening patiently probably subtracted a year or two from the average age I elicited from the young women and men I interviewed. This may well account for the younger age of first sexual awareness they reported when compared to previous research participants.[20]

What Is Remembered

Although some information is available about when individuals first experience same-sex attractions, much else mystifies us. Alfred Kinsey documented sources of erotic arousal, but few have followed up on his lead. How do the attractions change over time? What's remembered? What motivates the attractions? What are the contexts in which they first occur? Do any of these attractions vary in any systematic manner by age of first appearance, race or ethnicity of respondent, and social class or urban/rural upbringing of the individual? Do these experiences of same-sex attraction or desire have developmental implications—can they help us understand transitions to first sex, or enhance understanding of the teenager's sense of self?

One slight exception to this dearth of information is how adolescent girls and boys experience their first same-sex attractions. When young women and men are specifically asked to report their first awareness of same-sex desires, young women are far more likely to recall strong emotional bonds.[21] The average boy differs from the av-

126

erage girl more markedly in the recounting of the numerous, intense, distracting, and insistent sexual arousals he experiences—not once a week, but several times a day.[22] As one young man told me:

I couldn't not look because my penis was in a constant state of anti-droopiness. (Is that a word?) I always wanted to go swimming, but I'd just hang out in the locker room as long as I could and watch the guys come in, change clothes, go out, more come in, and I'd just sit there because I hated swimming but I loved going to swimming! Every day in the summer before first grade, and it was the high school guys who were my favorites because they'd flip each other with towels and grab each other and I'd just sit and watch. I'd have dry orgasms on the spot—they really exist, you know, although I learned in sex class that it's all so much myth and hype, but I'm your case study if you ever wanted someone to vouch for it.[23]

These differences in what is remembered can be found in the narratives of 200 Chicago-area youth during the late 1980s.[24] Gil Herdt and Andy Boxer succeeded in getting the teenagers to vividly recall their developmental histories. Though the teens reported having first sexual desires during their tenth year and their first same-sex fantasies a year later, many did not initially grasp the significance of their sexual desires, especially the sexual aspect. Boys "just happened" to look at and notice guys. Girls "just wanted" to be with a special girl. The targets of their desire were sometimes real people, sometimes celebrities, sometimes fictitious characters. Boys' sexual fantasies were more explicitly erotic than the girls'. One girl fantasized setting up a home with another girl with cars, cats, and no kids. One boy imagined having sex with several guys. Guilt for breaking a cultural taboo was often recalled. Maybe these teens' thoughts were forbidden, but they were nevertheless arousing.

Girls appear less likely to be exclusive in their attractions—that is, they experience arousal in response to both sexes. This difference has cross-cultural support. Both lesbians and gay males, however, tend to report homoerotic before heteroerotic attractions. They often recall the presence of memorable and intense same-sex erotic feelings within their ubiquitous, single-sex play groups.[25]

These sex differences have led some, including Anne Peplau, to hypothesize that female sexual attractions are more contextual than male attractions, and that they are more dependent on interpersonal relationships.[26] More central for young women is the desire for forming pair bonds, romantic intimacy, and emotional responsiveness. One young woman I interviewed recalled

these crushes I kept getting on teachers from the time I entered school. From kindergarten and first grade I was attracted to teachers, though I'm not sure it was sexual but was just there. I was the girl following the teacher around everywhere, in the classroom, in the bathroom, in the cafeteria, in the gym.

In fact, before even school, before kindergarten, I remember sitting under the piano in church on Wednesday nights and watching the gospel choir members practice because I had a crush on several of them. The way they moved, their joy, their flowing robes—I don't know, but just their presence made me love them.

Oh yes! I loved to brush my kindergarten teacher's hair, and I did it every time I could. I wonder if that meant something. I liked her a lot, and I cried when I left kindergarten—the only one to do so.[27]

This is not to deny that for "some women and in some social contexts, sexual orientation may be primarily about eroticism and sexuality."[28] Consider the recollections of this young woman, who can match any boy for explicit sexual memories:

Around four . . . I stole my dad's *Playboys* and looked at the cen-
terfolds. I always had sexual thoughts around women, and all
my fantasies were always about women. I asked this woman
friend of Mom's if I could squeeze her boobs (which were too
big to be real, silicon inflated I'm sure—she might even have
been a streetwalker) to see if they were real, and I did. I was four.
Then there was Wonder Woman! Damn! The source of my
childhood fantasies when I, you know, touched myself.[29]

To ignore intimacy and attachment as sexually central, however, is
to ignore the experience of most young women.[30] When asked what
they think causes sexual desire, young people clearly vary, depending
on their gender. College-age males endorsed biological processes and
a physical need for sex; females cited interpersonal experiences related to romantic love.[31]

Table 6.1 summarizes my findings on the contexts of the first
memories of childhood same-sex attractions.[32] From that table, it is
clear that traditional sex differences do emerge. The young women
are far more likely (six times as often) to remember an emotional attachment, while young men recount a sexual thought or arousal over
twice as often as girls. These contextual differences might help to explain the differences in timing between males and females. Crushes
tend to come later developmentally, during late childhood and early
adolescence, while sexual thoughts and arousal become apparent during early childhood games of house or doctor with best friends or
cousins. The data also suggest that a more nuanced perspective is in
order: some women recall sexual thoughts, and some men recall emotional contexts. Both sexes are equally likely to report sexual encounters. In the other contexts named in the table—over one third of all
responses—no sex differences are apparent.

Having so few case histories or narratives from contemporary
teens about their first sexual memories handicaps our understanding.

Table 6.1 Content of first memories of same-sex attraction

Content	Girls	Boys
Emotional attachment, infatuation, crush	40%	7%
General attractions, fascination	17%	20%
Sexual thoughts, dreams, arousal	15%	33%
Sexual behavior	13%	16%
Admiration or recognition of physical beauty	10%	17%
Desire to touch or feel	5%	7%

Source: Savin-Williams & Diamond, 2000.

These stories are rarely systematically collected, interpreted, and anchored in real-life events.

The Importance of What's Remembered

The young adults I interviewed tended not to be especially troubled as children by their same-sex desires. These feelings were understood to be simply a natural part of who they are. They may have been recognized as early as first memories or as late as the week before the interview. They may have consisted of a feeling of being different from peers, an admiration of the femininity or masculinity of same-sex peers, a sense of being sex atypical in behavior or interests, specific sexual encounters or the desire for them, a fascination with beauty or brawn, or just wanting to be held by another female or male.

The first memory might be an emotional, passionate infatuation toward a particular girl or boy or a series of girls or boys over a period of many years. It may involve stories of sexual exploits, dreams, and thoughts about best friends or cousins or movie stars or cartoon characters that were erotic and arousing then and perhaps still are today. The fact is, memories of same-sex attractions are recalled by those who feel different and those who do not, those who are teased and those who are not, popular girls and forgotten boys, girls who are "baby dykes" and then full-fledged lesbians and boys who question their sexuality and become "straight but curious."

Early attractions are often unrelated to when or what young adults eventually label themselves or disclose to others. They are also often unrelated to when one becomes involved in a romantic relationship (and with whom) and whether one ultimately has a positive or negative same-sex identity. Whether these attractions are general, specific, emotional, or sexual are similarly unrelated. They appear to stand alone, highly significant in the mind and experience of the girl or boy but unconnected to subsequent aspects of her or his sexuality.

As little as we know about the early sexuality of same-sex-attracted teens, it's huge by comparison to what we know about the early sexuality of heterosexual children and adolescents. This is both good and bad. It's good that we know at least something about the burgeoning sexuality of same-sex-attracted teenagers, but these explorations only of same-sex sexuality might deliver the message that it is in need of explanation and, some might add, justification. It is as if the sexual desires of heterosexuals have no onset, unique characteristics, or significance. Heterosexual arousal requires no exoneration or validation. It's just there—present since birth—prewired.

What can be said without equivocation is that early same-sex attractions for many teenagers are sources of great delight, fond remembrance, and lifetime reverberations; they may even be these individuals' most tender and pleasurable childhood memories. Although sexual desire can be disturbing and inexplicable, the bond between two girls or two boys feels natural, ultimately normal, and both arousing and soothing. Whether these same-sex feelings occur more often or are more intensely felt than for heterosexual children is unknown—and, perhaps in the end, unimportant.

If, however, same-sex-oriented young people experience more cross-orientation desire than heterosexual young people experience same-sex desire, it should not be surprising if they feel greater confusion during adolescence about the directionality of their sexual contacts and identity. The result may be a longer time to identify their sexuality, a larger number of misidentifications, and more fluidity in their identifications. Sexual encounters can be additional sources of information about one's sexual self. This is the subject of my next chapter.

7

First Sex

Childhood sexuality continues to be an enigma as we move from a consideration of sexual desires to actual sexual activity. The question for researchers is whether the sexual encounters of children and adolescents are meaningful when it comes to understanding their "mature" sexuality. In this chapter I review the limited information available on same-sex behavior among children and adolescents and the sexual behavior of adolescents who identify as gay, lesbian, or bisexual.

Based on extensive interviews with thousands of adults, Alfred Kinsey and his colleagues were the first to systematically explore the onset and nature of sexuality during childhood.[1] They argued that humans are naturally sexual and orgasmic throughout childhood and that their reluctance to engage in same-sex activities can often be attributable to repressive socialization that fails to acknowledge or tolerate such behavior. Despite these social predilections, many interviewees reported having orgasms prior to the onset of puberty, with sex play among same-sex peers being a principal source of erotic stimulation for both sexes.

These sex-play activities often consisted of exhibiting genitalia to friends and occasionally to strangers, and mutual touching among peers. Boys were more likely than girls to engage in sex play, primarily because boys, according to Kinsey and his colleagues, share an inherent interest in the "anatomy and functional capacities of male genitalia." Same-sex encounters among males declined from nearly two thirds of preadolescents to one quarter of early teens to one in ten older adolescents. As same-sex play declined, the ratio of heterosexual sex play increased because, according to Kinsey, teenagers became "heterosexually conditioned" and "continuously on the defensive against reactions which might be interpreted as homosexual."[2]

Among girls, same-sex play reached its peak at age nine and was as common as heterosexual sex play prior to age thirteen, but both types of activity were considerably less frequent among girls than among boys. By the onset of adolescence, one third of girls reported homosexual contact; this declined to one in ten during late adolescence. Girls preferred exhibitionism, genital examination, and manual manipulation of genitalia. Activities least common were inserting objects or fingers in the vagina and mouth-genital contact.[3]

Both boys and girls found these sexual encounters to be pleasurable and helpful in adding to their knowledge about sex, "private" body parts, masturbation, petting, sociosexual responses, and sexual techniques. Feelings of guilt could be the downside, especially if the children were reprimanded or punished by parents for their sexual exploration and interest. Kinsey found little evidence for the traditional view of childhood's being a time of sexual latency or arrest in sexual development. Although sharp pubertal increases in gonadal hormone levels corresponded to sharp increases in the intensity of self-reported sexual desires and activities, puberty was not an important developmental marker for the onset of sexual activities.

Several studies since Kinsey have documented children's "experiments with self-stimulation"—often in sex-positive cultures (for example, Scandinavian).[4] Apparently, children of both sexes and all sexual orientations exhibit a variety of solitary and partnered sexual behaviors. By age twelve, more than three fourths of Swedish high school students had engaged in autoerotic activities, including self-examination, self-stimulation, and viewing of sexually explicit pictures and/or videos.[5] Nearly twice as many boys as girls had masturbated and reached orgasm. Children in the United States appear to be less sexually adventurous, reporting far fewer instances of autoerotic activity. Perhaps the difference has to do with the fact that the U.S. researchers relied on the mothers' reports of their children's sexual behavior. Despite this fact, however, about one in three six- to twelve-year-olds were reported to "touch their sex parts at home."[6]

Like solitary sexual activities, partnered sex during childhood is seldom or under-documented. Almost half of young adult women and men in one study had interactive sex before they reached age six. In another sample, three quarters of both sexes had engaged in some form of sexual activity with a partner before age twelve.[7] Among the activities mentioned were talking about sex, kissing and hugging, watching or reading pornography (primarily boys), and humping or feigning intercourse. Sexually explicit activities—vaginal, anal, oral, and object intercourse—were reported by fewer than 5 percent of children. We don't know whether these are opposite- or same-sex activities because no one thinks (or dares) to ask children about the sex of their partner.

We also don't know the meaning or developmental relevance of childhood sexual activities—because no one asks. Regardless of gender of person and partner, if an early sexual contact is not abusive or coercive, then it likely has a positive impact on adolescent and adult sexual arousal, pleasure, satisfaction, and acceptance of various sexual behaviors for self and others.[8] Given the degree of sex negativity in U.S. culture, not all view these seemingly positive results as desirable outcomes. As for general social adjustment, sex among children is seldom associated with either developmental benefits or liabilities.[9]

To adequately understand the link between early sexual activities and adolescent physical, sexual, personal, and social development, we need to know more—about which children are having sex, in which contexts, what they are doing, and for what reasons. Given the inherent difficulties involved in conducting research on the sexual behavior of children, it may be some time before answers are forthcoming. Until then, at least one team of researchers has advised caution.[10] Although one might easily assume that children's sexual behaviors are "rehearsals" for pubertal and adult sexuality, no direct empirical data support this interpretation. For example, a significant number of heterosexual children engage in same-sex behavior. It is doubtful that this is rehearsal for adolescent homosexuality. Maybe it's a "test" for whether they prefer boys or girls. Or maybe it's just a chance to have fun.

Childhood sexual activity may be an altogether different phenomenon from adolescent sexual activity, with its own developmentally specific motives, qualities, and functions that correspond to a child's social, cognitive, and biological maturation. Unfortunately, few have explored these possibilities, despite reports of teenagers who distinguish their "early sex when I was a kid" from their adolescent "real sex" experiences. This distinction was actually noted—but then dropped—in the first empirical study of gay youth.[11] The majority of the young gay male respondents described engaging in early, prepubertal sexual experiences, mutual body exploration, and curiosity-based sex play. They were emphatic, however, about making "a distinction between merely having sexual contact with another male and actually having a homosexual experience."

Most likely, Kinsey was right. Sexuality develops gradually over the course of childhood through a subtle and gradual intertwining of physical and social experiences. Children become aroused in response to erotic stimuli, frequently during play activities with their friends. Although the traditional view is that most children do not act on sexual feelings until puberty, the supposed exceptions seem to rule. Why? Perhaps because it's fun. The possibility that children have an additional (unconscious) motivation for their same-sex encounters or that sex might have a meaning or significance for their personal identity is, at least for now, more fantasy than established fact.

As for adolescents who engage in same-sex contact, one of two interpretations is usually offered: either they are simply experimenting and will eventually identify as heterosexual, or they are gay and are explicitly or covertly expressing their homosexuality. Complicating these seemingly sensible assertions, however, are data that caution against simple and universal conclusions and in favor of a differential developmental trajectories perspective. For example, consider the following:

- Not all same-sex-attracted teenagers are sexually active and are thus heterosexually and homosexually virgins.
- Some teens only have cross-orientation sex—that is, some are gay virgins but heterosexually experienced and some are heterosexual virgins but homosexually experienced.
- Most same-sex-attracted teens and an unknown number of heterosexual ones have sex with both girls and boys.
- Some young people, regardless of sexual orientation, have only same-sex or opposite-sex encounters.

The proportion of gay virgins—defined as not having "sex" with a same-sex partner—among those who identify as gay is usually below 10 percent for boys and 20 percent for girls. The reasons for these young people being virgins are the same reasons heterosexual young people give—physical and emotional immaturity, lack of opportunity, religious prohibition, social awkwardness, and personal values.

Boys, for example, have had the following to say:

"I'm looking for someone very special, but it is really hard to meet such a guy. They all just want sex. I need to know the person; ideally we would be friends for a while. This I know is an elusive goal but I want to hold onto it."[12]

"I was a late bloomer and so in junior high school I had no real sexual orgasms . . . I guess I've never felt the need for sex, although I would like to try it sometime."[13]

"I knew I was attracted to boys in my class but I couldn't be gay because of all the horrible stuff that was associated with it. Me, a good kid, just could not be all of that. To stick it up someone's ass . . ."[14]

"I'm just not a sexual person and don't have sex with random people. I want to feel something first and know it is going to be a long-term relationship."[15]

By contrast to previous research, an Internet survey of same-sex-attracted teens found that nearly 30 percent of young men and 50 percent of young women reported that they have not had sex with a same-sex partner. What is significant about this study is that many of those respondents did not identify as gay; they only had to have same-sex attractions to participate. This suggests that the proportion of non–gay-identified same-sex-attracted teens who have not had gay sex might be larger than the proportion of gay-identified teens who have not had gay sex.[16]

These Internet data confirm other investigations that boys are more likely than girls to report same-sex pursuits and that girls are more likely than boys to engage in heterosexual activities.[17] An Australian study provides cross-cultural support for these findings. Girls said they more often exclusively engaged in sex with boys than with girls or with both sexes.[18] Boys were more exclusively same-sex focused. Indeed, only a minority of gay-identified teens engages solely in same-sex behavior, and some gay teens have a considerable amount of cross-orientation sex.[19] A study based on students in Massachusetts public schools found that gay students were four times more likely than heterosexual students to have sexual intercourse before age thirteen and twice as likely to have had sexual intercourse.[20]

Given cultural heterocentrism and active sexual prejudice, it is not surprising that most adolescents who have had same-sex encounters claim to be heterosexual.[21] With the dearth of longitudinal research, it is impossible to know for certain what proportion of adolescent same-sex activity represents experimentation, what proportion represents an expression of adolescent same-sex orientation, and what proportion springs from some other motivation.

When?

One near-unanimous truth is that gay boys report an earlier age for first having sex with another boy than girls report sex with another girl. The average gay boy first has sex with a same-sex partner shortly after the onset of puberty, at the age of thirteen or fourteen. (I'll leave aside for now the question of what constitutes gay sex.) For the average lesbian girl, it's at least a year or two later. The reverse is true, however, for the onset of first heterosexual contact among teens with predominantly same-sex desires. A young lesbian, on average, has first sex with a boy when she is twelve or thirteen years old. A young gay man has sex with a girl a few years later. One result of these patterns is that a young gay man's first sex is usually with a boy rather than a girl, while a young lesbian's first sexual experience is also with a boy.[22] For example, among Chicago youth, Gil Herdt and Andy Boxer reported that girls were twice as likely as boys to have heterosexual and then gay sex and half as likely to have an exclusively gay sexual pattern.[23]

Given that these are average ages, many exceptions exist. Age of first sexual encounters ranges from early childhood (age five or six years is not uncommon) to the age of the oldest participant. Because her single mother was often at work, one young woman I interviewed recalled being able to have friends over. This included her best friend, Ashley, with whom she reported engaging in sexual activity:

We were both eight and it was penetration of each other with our fingers—this one, the big one. We had been best friends for

139

several years and our play just naturally went this way. We didn't understand anything about sex or anything.

I cared for her like I did for all my friends, but I did not love her in any special way. It was play sex. Fondling and kissed a lot. We weren't lovers, just experimenters. Continued for six months until she told her aunt and then we had to give it up. Very little contact since. She is married with three children.[24]

By contrast, another young woman waited many years after she first recognized her same-sex sexuality for her maiden sexual adventure:

At nineteen I went to this folk festival by myself in Vancouver and I saw this woman three years older and we started talking. Didn't kiss. I called her after I got back home and we got together and then we kissed. I spent the week with her and so I guess we had sex on our second date although it was a couple of weeks after the first. This was after I came out.[25]

More evidence is provided by Tony D'Augelli. His "Challenges and Coping Project" recruited 350 young people from fifty-nine community-based gay organizations and college gay groups throughout the United States.[26] Although the definition of sexual behavior was not specified—the question being simply about "sexual experiences with males/females"—the results are congruent with those of other studies (see Table 7.1).

Why should both same-sex-attracted girls and boys tend to have their first sex with a boy?[27] Is it that boys are more readily available? Less complicated? Is it that girls are less aware that their attractions to girls are sexual and not just emotionally intimate?

The initial heterosexual experience for both same-sex-attracted girls and boys usually occurs within the context of a dating relationship. Given this, the tendency for girls to have an opposite- before a same-sex encounter likely reflects the greater social pressures on

Table 7.1   Sexual behavior of D'Augelli respondents

	Females	Males
Same-sex sexual contact		
Incidence	86%	95%
Mean age	15.9	14.3
Age range of first encounter	8–21 years	5–20 years
Opposite-sex sexual contact		
Incidence	79%	42%
Mean age	13.3	14.4
Age range of first encounter	3–21 years	8–19 years

Source: D'Augelli, 1998.

teenage girls than boys to date, the greater likelihood that girls will bo the "invitee" rather than the "inviter" in arranging the date, and the greater tendency for women to be authentically attracted to both sexes.[28]

One young woman I interviewed had begun her sexual career with a boy she started dating at soccer camp. After the first week he initiated sex. She recalled:

We both wanted this. We kissed and he touched my breast and then touched below the waist in a steady progression. I tried to jerk him off and he tried to go down on me. Not successful! It was goal-oriented fooling around.

It was the first of six times during the three-week soccer camp. More like groping in the dark than real sex because no one came. It felt funny because we thought we knew what we were doing. It didn't progress much beyond this point. When we got back from camp it was over. We were so cute but it was so boring, ugh![29]

Perhaps the real arbitrator is the girl. She is more circumspect and discriminating when it comes to sexual activity and thus more likely to postpone sex regardless of whether the suitor is another girl (easier to postpone because the prospective partner has the same point of reference) or a boy (more difficult because the boy is usually older, holds out the promise of prestige, and may be more persistent).

It is difficult to detect from these studies what provokes one girl or boy to engage in early same-sex encounters, even prior to adrenarche, while another becomes sexually involved only after all biological markers of pubescence are long past. In both very early and very late cases, psychosocial events likely take precedence over biological factors as motivating forces. It will happen given the right alignment of congruent circumstances or "accidents"—a willing cousin or friend sleeping over, a night when parents are out for dinner, the message some young people vividly recall to "take a chance on life," the food, the lighting, the music, the drugs.

One final observation: same-sex-attracted girls are having sex with boys and girls earlier than in previous generations (and more often!). Oddly enough, there has been no comparable historic trend for gay-identified boys' first sex with a boy.[30] Given the fact that all other developmental milestones have shown a steady decrease in onset age, this aberration begs explaining. Perhaps the motivating forces for having first gay sex have not changed for boys. The biological spur of puberty, the availability of male partners, and the tacit social approval boys receive that it's okay to pursue sexual pleasure are factors that have remained relatively steady across generations. Whatever the reason, boys for generations have engaged in sexual activities with other boys at about the same age.

With Whom?

Researchers and public-health officials over the past two decades or more have been very interested in the number of sexual partners gay boys have, because of the risk associated with HIV and AIDS. After reading the first study ever conducted on gay youth, many of whom were hustlers and prostitutes, the idea that young homosexual males had many sex partners seemed to be confirmed. One eighteen-year-old in that study reported having over 3,000 male sexual partners. This number was obtained by his spending every weekend for three years in public restrooms, where he fellated men. The median number of male partners in the study was 50. There were plenty of female sex partners, too. Almost one quarter of the boys reported having more than 10 female partners.[31]

Few investigators since have come close to duplicating these numbers—unless the young men were recruited from similar sources. One such subject might be a New York City youth seeking the services of the Hetrick-Martin community-based recreational and social services agency. The average male caller or visitor there reported having 69 male and 7 female partners. Double these numbers for the average number of sexual *encounters*.[32]

Using the same male population but moving forward nearly two decades to the 1990s, Margaret Rosario and her colleagues report far fewer lifetime male (14) and female (4) partners, but not fewer sexual encounters. This might well reflect the AIDS scare and a willingness on the part of the young male respondents to forego anonymous, causal sex without having to give up the frequency with which they have sex.[33] Other samples have shown the number of lifetime sexual partners among adolescent boys to be even lower. Is this the impact of recruitment venue—fewer support groups and more college organizations? So it would seem. Tony D'Augelli reported a median of 6 lifetime same-sex partners among college males, with a range from 0 to 50. [34] Consistently, across studies, young men with a large number of male sex partners are the same ones who have a substantial number of female sex partners. In a study of students in Vermont public schools, boys with five or more male partners nearly always had two or more female partners.[35]

Although far less is documented about the sexual activities of same-sex-attracted young women,[36] they have seldom chalked up the extreme number of partners that their gay brothers have done. They have fewer lifetime female (8) and male (6) partners than young gay men, but they have far more sexual encounters with their female (420) and male (103) partners. It would appear that young women may be forgoing casual sexual relationships, but they are not abstaining from sexual contact. They're maintaining a sexual relationship with their sex partners for a long time and having considerable sex as a result.[37]

As for what actually happens when two adolescents have same-sex sex, we are not sure. Who would dare ask?

What?

Determining which adolescents have had sex, at what age, and with how many sex partners largely depends on which behaviors are deemed "sexual." Usually it's a version of the generic question "Have you had sexual intercourse/experience with a male/female?" Without elaboration or probes, it is next to impossible for a respondent to know exactly which behaviors should be counted.[38] Definitions of sex vary according to the sexual identity status and the gender of the young person. Nearly all gay college men in one study viewed penile-anal intercourse as sex. Somewhat fewer found oral-genital contact (80 percent), use of sex accessories (65 percent), and oral-anal contact (60 percent) to count as having sex. Nearly all gay women, by contrast, considered oral-genital contact and use of sex accessories as sex; they were somewhat less inclined to see hand-genital contact (80 percent) and oral-anal contact (70 percent) as sex. Some particular activities, especially deep kissing and touching breasts, gay men were more likely than lesbians to call "sex." Other activities, especially oral and manual stimulation of genitals, same-sex-attracted women were more inclined to define as sex. One in ten young gay men viewed deep kissing as sex. Two in ten said an orgasm was necessary—twice the rate as for young gay women. Heterosexual college students didn't necessarily agree with these definitions of sex.[39]

When these various sexual behaviors first occur differs among individuals and across the sexes. Responding to a sexual risk assessment questionnaire, young women reported having their first manual (hand-genital) contact with another female when they averaged age thirteen. It was age fourteen for their first oral, anal, and oral-anal female contact.[40] Among young gay men, the age spread among types of sex was broader. Boys averaged age twelve for first manual sex, but nearly age fifteen for anilingus.

How many gay teens have had sex also depends on what is being referenced.[41] Nearly nine in ten adolescent gay boys have had manual and oral sex with another male. Only about half, however, have engaged in oral-anal contact. If being the passive partner in male-male anal sex counts as more sexual than being the active partner, then more adolescent boys have had sex. If heterosexual sex for girls is considered to be manual and penile-vaginal contact with boys, then sex was far more common than if anal sex was the criterion. Both male and female gay respondents were as likely to be an active as a receptive partner in manual or oral sex when the partner is a male. When the partner is a female, females were more likely than males to be the active partner.

The timing of what type of sexual activity occurs during adolescence clearly depends on whether the partner referenced is a girl or a boy, as illustrated in Table 7.2.[42] Thus, what matters is not only the specific behavior that counts as sex but also the sex of the partner.

Table 7.2   Timing of sexual behavior

Rank order	Female-female	Male-male	Female-male
Earliest	Oral	Oral	Oral
Early	Vaginal-digital	Anal	Vaginal-digital
Middle	Anilingus	Anilingus	Vaginal-penile
Late	Vaginal-dildo	Anal-dildo	Anal
Latest	Anal-dildo		Anal-dildo

Source: Rosario et al., 1999.

145

Table 7.3   Internet survey of sexual behavior

	% of girls			% of boys		
Sexual behavior	Lesbian	Bi	Unsure	Gay	Bi	Unsure
Received same-sex oral	50	39	13	66	66	39
Gave same-sex oral	48	35	15	68	67	37
Received cross-sex oral	34	52	43	16	43	22
Gave cross-sex oral	35	54	38	9	35	16
Received same/cross-sex anal	7	18	6	42	40	17
Gave same-sex anal				41	40	17
Gave cross-sex anal				1	11	1
Vaginal with sex toy	18	18	6			
Penile/vaginal intercourse				14	41	19

Source: Kryzan, 1997.

One point seldom addressed is whether the incidence, prevalence, sequence, or onset age of sex varies depending on an adolescent's degree of same-sex sexuality. For example, does a girl totally committed to same-sex sexuality have a particular sex act at a younger age than a girl only peripherally interested in sex with another girl? An Internet survey, summarized in Table 7.3, suggests that the proportion of same-sex-attracted young people who engage in particular sex acts depends on the sex of the partner, the behavior referenced, *and* the sexual identity of the young woman or man.[43]

Take oral sex as an example. It is the most common same-sex activity among both young women and men, both of whom are as likely to give as to receive, regardless of their sexual identity. However, the proportion who have had oral sex drops when the partner is an opposite-sex partner, especially precipitously among gay males (from two thirds to one sixth). Gay boys rarely give girls oral sex.

Also, bisexuals of both sexes have some similarities to their gay sisters and brothers, but they also differ. The proportion of gay and bisexual boys who have had oral or anal sex with another male is virtually the same. However, when it comes to receiving and giving oral sex with a female and engaging in vaginal sex, bisexual boys are three to four times more likely to have had sex than gay boys. Similar but less pronounced differences are apparent among lesbian and bisexual girls.

A study of college women in the 1970s provides more information. Of the 160 college women in the study, 10 percent reported that they had sex with a woman.[44] The most common activities, from most to least prevalent, were nude kissing and caressing without genital contact, manual genital contact, mutual pubic rubbing, and cunnilingus. Nearly all the women in this study had intercourse with a man, often prior to having sex with a woman. Compared to collegiate women without same-sex contact, the women in this study:

had half as many male partners
had their first sexual experience nearly two years later
had a narrower range of sexual activities with men
were half as likely to "almost always" have an orgasm with a man
were more likely to have had sex with a man they did not love
were half as likely to usually enjoy fellatio with a man
were four times more likely to masturbate regularly and to enjoy it
were far less likely to have had their most pleasurable orgasm during intercourse with a man
were more likely to fantasize during sex
were more likely to want daily sex

The most valuable information is in the details. The degree, proportion, and level of sex most clearly distinguished the women who did and did not have sex with a woman. Yes, women who had sex with women also had sex with men. But they had it less often, they had it later, and they enjoyed it less.

Whether these differences remain true today is unknown, in part because researchers appear to be reluctant to ask adolescents specifically what they do when they have sex and whether they enjoyed it. Even less is known about the context and motivation for sex.

Where and Why?

We probably shouldn't make too much of the findings reported so far in this chapter because so little is known about the meaning or significance for the young person of these initial forays into sex. The motives and contexts for the first same-sex experience are little understood.

For children's same-sex activities, the most common context is play with best friends, cousins, and occasionally a sibling or older known person. Motives often include curiosity and pleasure—these are fun encounters without much meaning. The primary drawback is fear of parental punishment. Partners are usually perceived to be heterosexual, and the sex is either a single event or activities that occur over many years. In retrospect, respondents think that they might have been more "into it" than their partners.[45] One girl recalled:

We were playing house and pretending to have sex. So [there was] some rubbing our genitals together. Kissing, but could not do it on the lips. Genitalia touching, dry sex, rubbing. And with two other girls as well later on. Me always wanting more of it than them.

I always ached to play these games but knew I shouldn't because they were wrong. Was this because of my emotional void? Something you can get from a girl you can't from a boy. Physical desire? Because it felt so good. To be different? I was always the rebel.

It is likely, but not documented, that heterosexual children also engage in these childhood same-sex play activities for the same reasons and with the same reservations. Few, however, mention same-sex activities when talking with researchers, parents, or mental health professionals. Perhaps the activities were forgotten because they seemed of such little significance; or they were not defined as sexual, even when genital contact occurred; or the respondents failed to assign meaning to them. One gay young man I interviewed believed that his first same-sex partner really was straight, and that the sex they had at summer camp was an experiment for one and the real thing for the other:

Then when we got home he lost interest because he didn't want to do it anymore, but I did. It was clearly more than just an experiment for me. He got me to promise that "let's never talk about it," but I wanted to and *I* knew that I wasn't supposed to.

After this in high school he only went out with girls and seemed really sex obsessed. I heard once that he asked guys for blow jobs, to give him one but he never touched them. He's married and got four kids. I see him around occasionally. I don't know what he'd say about our summer camp "experiments."[46]

Similar to what we know about heterosexual sexual activities, same-sex-attracted girls tend to engage in their first sex with a female within the context of a friendship or a dating relationship (two thirds in one study). [47] Some boys also prefer "relationship sex" (one third in the same study), although their most common context for first sex is as a purely physical encounter.

Sometimes, however, this difference between boys and girls is overemphasized. The fact is, adolescent boys also like relationship sex. One qualitative study found that more young women than men had stable same-sex relationships, had few sex partners, and attached emotional, romantic meaning to their relationships prior to sex.[48] As expected, young men more frequently found sex partners by cruising strangers. *However*, they most preferred sex with friends and relatives.[49] Even at-risk adolescent boys had sex three times more often with same-age friends than with older strangers.

The reverse is also seldom acknowledged. Some adolescent girls do not shun anonymous sex. An Internet survey posed the question

"Would you likely have sex with someone you just met and would never see again?"[50] Half of the young men responded "yes/maybe," and nearly four in ten of the young women also replied in the affirmative. This finding does not indicate a huge difference between the sexes. Although young women of all sexual orientations are more likely than young men to have, and perhaps prefer, sex within a known relationship, this is only a matter of degree, not of kind.[51]

Besides the nature of the sex partner, age has also been a topic of some concern. The belief—or fear—is that young people are sexually abused by an older person and hence are led into same-sex sexuality. Though it is true that the first male partner of a young man tends to be six years older on average, the first female partner of a young woman is overwhelmingly similar in age (within three years). The reverse characterizes the first heterosexual partner. A young man tends to be close in age to his first female partner (within two years), while a young woman tends to be three years younger than her first male partner.[52]

Similar trends, but with smaller age differences, are reported in an Internet survey. Nearly three quarters of all sex partners, for young gay women and men alike, were found to be within two years of each other. When the partner is more than six years older (this is the case with 20 percent of the young men and 10 percent of the young women), it is nearly always a male partner.[53] If an adolescent of either gender with same-sex attractions has an older sex partner, the issue is not one of sexual orientation but the fact that the sex partner is likely to be male. It's also worth noting that same-sex-attracted young people almost never (less than 2 percent in the study just cited) have a sex partner who is three or more years younger. That is, they are not "sexually abusing" children.

These findings are consistent with the first and third tenets of a differential developmental trajectories perspective: that is, the sexual behavior of same-sex-attracted teens is more similar to the sexual behavior of heterosexual adolescents of their own sex than it is to the behavior of same-sex-attracted teens of the opposite sex; and the sexes are not opposite in their sexuality but overlap in many significant ways. Gil Herdt and Andy Boxer agree; they note, "In general, boys attached more emphasis to sexual pleasure, while the girls viewed emotional closeness as more important. But the boys also clearly express needs for emotional closeness, and lesbian youth certainly did not disregard sexual pleasure."[54]

Herdt and Boxer also included a question in their study that is seldom asked of research participants' sexual behavior: Was the sex good or was it bad?

How Was It?

On a scale of 1 (very bad) to 5 (very good), the Chicago young people studied by Herdt and Boxer rated their first same-sex experience as 3.6—better than average and considerably higher than their first heterosexual experience, which they rated at 2.8. Even at this rating, however, heterosexual sex was found to be almost "average."[55] In another survey of same-sex-attracted youth, over half evaluated their first sexual experience (unstated but likely same-sex) as positive. About one quarter believed it was negative or that they were taken advantage of. Bisexuals had the most positive first experience, while questioning and unsure young adults of both sexes had the least positive first experiences.[56]

It's not unusual for teens with same-sex desires to feel that both their first gay and straight sex experiences are deeply satisfying, sometimes only emotionally, sometimes only physically, but sometimes both emotionally and physically.[57] I assume this would also characterize the first gay and straight sex of heterosexual youth, though we do not know this for certain because relevant data have yet to be collected.

Sexual Behavior: A Complex Subject

A simple knowledge of the specific activities involved in adolescent sexuality is of little value. Feelings, fantasies, attractions, desires, and meaning are so intertwined with sexual behavior that what we think we know about young people and sex would be laughable if it weren't so wrong.[58] That, however, must remain the subject of another book. Here, I'll simply give a sense of how complex the subject of sex can be by noting a study that simply divided same-sex-attracted respondents into two groups, gay/lesbian and bisexual, and then distinguished whether they had ever identified as the other group (if so, they were said to be "transitional" as opposed to "stable").[59] The findings regarding number of sex partners and age of initiating sex are summarized for each sex (rather than by sexual orientation), followed by my brief interpretation in parentheses.

GIRLS

- Compared to their lesbian classmates, bisexual girls had fewer lifetime female partners (1 versus 4) but more male partners (5 versus 3). They did not differ on age of first sex with either girls or boys. (These findings are to be expected, given that bisexual girls tend to be more male- and less female-oriented than lesbians, but why aren't these findings reflected in age of first sex? Perhaps socialization pressures are operating to determine these data.)
- Although stable and transitional lesbians did not differ in age of first sex with males or females or number of female partners, those who changed their label from bisexual to lesbian had more male partners. (These are the girls who probably have stronger male attractions than those who never doubted their lesbian identity. Again, the differences are not reflected in the

data on age of first sex. The number of female partners might be equal because the transitional lesbians "caught up.")

- Those who changed from lesbian to bisexual had more female partners than stable bisexuals, but did not differ in age of first sex with males or females or number of male partners. (These girls may have stronger same-sex attractions, which leads them to have more sex with girls than those who always knew they were attracted to both sexes. Again, age of first sex does not differ.)

- Age of initiating first sex with a female or male appears unrelated to current or historic identity patterns. However, the number and distribution of sex partners do differ, with the number of male partners distinguishing transitional from stable lesbians and number of female partners distinguishing transitional from stable bisexuals. (One fascinating question not explored in this study is whether bisexual-to-lesbian girls vary from lesbian-to-bisexual girls on any domain. My guess is that the differences are subtle and are more experiential than biologically based.)

BOYS

- Gay-identified boys were no more likely than their bisexual classmates to have male partners (5), but they had more sex with these partners and they had fewer female partners (0 versus 3). (This is consistent with the literature that the critical factor is less the number of male partners—who are readily available—than the number of female partners. Bisexuals, who are more strongly motivated to have sex with girls, will be more likely than gays to find female partners.)

- Bisexual-to-gay boys had both more female and more male partners than those who never doubted their gay status. (The surprising finding here is that the bisexual-to-gay boys have more male partners than the stable gay boys. One possibility is that the former needs more "proof "—that is, male partners—to make the transition from bisexual to gay. Another possibility is that they have a higher libido.)

- Considering the two bisexual subgroups, the gay-to-bisexual boys had more male partners than did the stable bisexuals, but the two groups did not differ on number of female sex partners. (The greater number of male sex partners makes sense for the gay-to-bisexual boys if in the process of discovering their identity they rely more on readily available male sex partners. However, they apparently did not forsake sexual encounters with girls.)

- Similar to girls, age of initiating first sex with either gender did not distinguish identity status or patterns. Rather, it was the number of sex partners that differentiated the various patterns. Boys who started out as bisexual— whether they remained in this category or transitioned to gay—tended to have more female partners. Boys who started out as gay likewise had more male partners, true to their same-sex attractions. Regardless of outcome, those who transitioned had more male partners than those who remained stable. (This may indicate the importance of the availability of male partners for "experimentation." As for the girls, a comparison of the two transitional groups would be informative for addressing these issues.)

Clearly, in order to understand adolescent sexuality it's beneficial to examine degree of same-sex attraction, the development of these attractions, and individuals' history of sexual identity labels. Unfortunately, we know relatively little about all of these things.

This chapter, in short, illustrates what has yet to be known about same-sex sexuality more than what is known.[60] The question for same-sex-attracted young people as they sort through their feelings of differentness, their gender expression, their initial same-sex attractions, and their sexual encounters with both girls and boys is whether any of this means anything about who they are.

8

Identity

When an adolescent has strong and persistent same-sex attractions, she or he might or might not also feel different, display sex-atypical behavior or interests, and engage in same-sex behavior. Alternatively, she or he may have such feelings and behavior and feel no same-sex attractions.

Disagreement over what is supposed to predict or characterize gayness might cause a young person to doubt whether she or he is gay or wonder if perhaps she or he is. The progression from feeling different in early childhood to having same-sex attractions in late childhood to engaging in gay sex in early adolescence happens to some, but clearly not all, teens. The ones who conform to this pattern may be those most likely to identify as gay during middle adolescence. They have a script, and their life seems to follow it. Many others, however, don't label their sexuality because parts of their script just don't seem to fit. One young woman, for example, had this to say:

The question is "Who am I attracted to?" I've said a bunch of times, "I'm a lesbian," and would then say, "Nope." But I'm not outgrowing it and I'm not twelve anymore. I was in a small liberal arts college and was encouraged to explore, and I didn't. There were professors on the spectrum and I knew that. When it is intense I don't know what to do about it. Should I try to do something or ignore it? There are weeks when I don't think about it. I'm looking at women more and I'm more attracted to them. With guys mostly I dismiss them but some I can get intense about, but I can get intense with women, too. I can't act on it because I'm in a relationship with a guy. With guys for me it's not physical as much as intellectual and their personality.[1]

Sexual identity stage theorists, naturally enough, have a lot to say about these issues. According to Vivienne Cass, individuals accept that their sexual feelings, actions, or thoughts might be labeled "homosexual" during Stage 2 and progress to the belief that they are probably homosexual at the beginning of Stage 3. By the conclusion of Stage 3, they are certain about it but do not fully accept the idea; that happens at Stage 4. By the conclusion of Stage 4, they will have developed a positive image of themselves as homosexual and will feel comfortable among other homosexuals.[2]

For Richard Troiden, individuals keep separate their "consciousness of sexual feelings" from any sense of a sexual identity during Stage 2. That is, they acknowledge their sexual feelings and behavior as "undeniable" yet believe that these feelings have very little if anything to do with what they are. They do not attribute a name or an identity to their sexuality until they label themselves as homosexual at the beginning of Stage 3. Later, they become involved in the homosexual subculture and ultimately come to define homosexuality as a positive and viable lifestyle.[3]

Whether any teenager actually follows these patterns is unknown. I have my doubts. Certainly the supposed patterns must vary by gender, ethnicity, personality characteristics, income level, and generation. Can they possibly be true for all contemporary teenagers? In my interviews with young adults, I found that gender made a huge difference in developmental progression. Young men were far more likely than women to recall a time when they said to themselves, "Hey, I know I'm attracted to other guys [or girls in the case of young women], but that doesn't mean I'm gay!" Young women were more apt to tell me, "As soon as I realized what sex I was attracted to, I knew what I was."

Many contemporary teens of various sexualities—not just gay teenagers—question their sexual identity. Some ultimately determine their sexual identity. Others do not.

Questioning

Nearly every one of the adult men Richard Troiden interviewed for his dissertation recalled a time when they questioned their sexuality.[4] What most often led to their questioning was their having a sexual experience with another male. Others were led to questioning because they felt sexually aroused by a male, because they learned about homosexuality and realized that it might apply to them, or because they weren't being turned on by women. Rarely were they led to question their sexuality because they developed a crush on another male (though this, too, occasionally happened).

One young man I interviewed contended that he knew he wasn't gay, except for when he thought too much about the gay sex he was having. He questioned his sexuality, but he wasn't quite ready to say the word "gay" about himself. He recalled:

> In junior high I knew that what I was doing with boys might be called homosexual sex, but because I found girls really attractive and was also having sex with them then I knew that I could not be gay because fags didn't have sex with girls, didn't wrestle, didn't like sports, and didn't like guy things, which was all of what I was.[5]

Lisa Diamond reports that what provokes young women's first sexual questioning is rarely a sexual arousal or experience but feelings of attraction for other women and developing an emotional crush or attachment to another woman. Another factor is exposure to a facilitating environment, such as taking women studies college courses or having conversations with friends about gay issues.[6]

One young woman I interviewed, who was a track and basketball star, found love on the other side of the court during a college scrimmage game. She remembers the exact date and her feelings:

I felt an overwhelming attraction toward her that I never had before, and I said that this is it. I had experiences before but none so overwhelming. I struggled with this for a long time.

A crush on the girl I was competing against! This hit me really hard, and I could hardly play all night. So I broke up with my boyfriend and asked myself, "What's going on?!"

I never denied it to myself but I never had acknowledged before my crush. I'd have these crazy dreams about women, once I almost kissed a woman, but I never thought about their meaning. I thought about it but I had no gay culture or idea what it meant to be a lesbian.[7]

Why the questions? Why not just assume one is gay and move on? Why should a teen assume that her attraction for another woman is just a phase or less real or just a "tendency"? Troiden's men said they couldn't tolerate the possibly that they might be homosexual because they were so unlike "real" homosexuals. They had certain images of how homosexuals looked, how homosexuals acted, how homosexuals had sex. It wasn't them. Others denied the obvious because they had not yet had gay sex, which for them constituted the real proof of homosexuality. Even some who had had sex with other boys interpreted it as merely sexual release, thinking that it meant nothing about their future lifestyle. These respondents of Troiden's, however, were men who came of age in the 1950s. Whether such beliefs are characteristic of the sexual questioning of contemporary teens is unknown, but perhaps likely.

One contemporary study that touched on these issues recruited young people from urban community-based social and recreational agencies.[8] Over 80 percent considered at some point in their development that they "might be gay/lesbian/bisexual"—which may be taken as an indication of sexual questioning. Boys recalled having these thoughts at the average age of twelve; girls, a year later. What caused this questioning during early adolescence? Unfortunately, this issue wasn't investigated. Many of the respondents recalled having same-sex attractions, fantasies, and arousal to erotica at an earlier age, ten to twelve years. These may have motivated their sexual questioning. Although the pairing of sexual motives and questioning is not unusual,[9] we don't know if the two things are connected with each other or if they influence the development of a sexual identity.

When ages for sexual questioning are given, they are nearly always averages, and the ages given are usually in early adolescence. Yet the range can be quite broad—starting before the magical age of ten. Urban support group members were asked, "When did you first realize that you were homosexual?" Girls and boys were evenly split into three age groups: childhood (four to ten years), early adolescence (eleven to thirteen), and adolescence (fourteen to seventeen).[10] The average might be "early adolescence," but this age category represents only a minority of the teens.

I found sex differences in my interviews with young adults. Yes, early adolescence was the prime time during which young men recalled having "homosexual" or "gaylike" attractions or qualities but were not yet willing to label themselves as gay persons. Young women were less likely to remember such a time but, if they did, it was late puberty, averaging age fifteen years. At the extremes, for both sexes, were individuals who named their attractions but not themselves at age six. Others waited until young adulthood to make the connection—and several young women I talked with were yet to make the association. Because they were so exceedingly "weird" or so out of the mainstream as a teenager, they believed their attraction to women was simply another manifestation of their strangeness. It signified their rebellious, outsider status, not their sexuality.

Adopting a Sexual Identity

A few early adolescents connect their questioning with their sexual identity, but for most it has to wait until their high school years. Those who acknowledge their identity early simultaneously realize the inevitable and the obvious. One young woman asserted that she never had a questioning phase: "As soon as I heard the term [lesbian] I realized it was me."[11] Why hers was a seamless transition and others' are not is unknown. Perhaps her sexuality was felt so intensely that she could not ignore its meaning. Or perhaps one's experiences, such as discovering a friend is gay or falling madly in love with someone, inspire early adoption of a sexual identity.

FROM QUESTIONING TO IDENTIFYING

The transition that leads to sexual questioning does not necessarily parallel the transition to a same-sex identity. Gil Herdt and Andy Boxer suggest that the second might simply be a matter of "self-dialogue"—a reflective, internal process by which one recognizes and then accepts same-sex desires.[12] Perhaps. However, the first two gay-youth studies ever conducted suggest that the evolution from a "maybe" to a "likely" to a "certainly" to a "proudly" gay person is powered by sex, at least among boys. Nearly all young men in one study reported that they had a homosexual experience to orgasm prior to concluding "I am a homosexual."[13] This may also be true among contemporary teenagers.[14]

Factors other than sex also influence sexual labeling. Twice as important as having gay sex to the point of orgasm, even among gay boys, are persistent attractions to men.[15] Also mentioned are the lack

Table 8.1 Content involved in self-labeling

Content	Girls	Boys
Emotional attachment, infatuation, crush	25%	15%
General attractions, fascination	20%	18%
Facilitative book, movie, course, program	20%	9%
Friends	10%	13%
Sexual thoughts, dreams, arousal	9%	26%
Admiration or recognition of physical beauty	8%	0%
Lack of interest in other sex	6%	7%
Same-sex sexual contact	2%	13%

Source: Savin-Williams, 1998a, in preparation; Savin-Williams & Diamond, 2000.

of attraction to women, the fact that the sex they have with women is less intense, and an identification with a gay community. For bisexual boys, persistent attractions to both sexes is critical. Three quarters of an Australian sample of both girls and boys nominated same-sex attraction as the most compelling agent for recognition of their gay identity.[16] Same-sex fantasies were endorsed by two thirds, an assertion that they "just knew" by over half, and a sexual experience by half.

Among the young adults I interviewed, open-ended responses of what led to a self-label were grouped into eight categories (see Table 8.1). Young women frequently recalled the significance of an emotional attachment or crush and the facilitative role of a special book, college course, or movie. A same-sex experience was not on their radar screen. Young men, by contrast, typified prior research. Sex was very important to them. What was least important for both was lack of other-sex interest and pure physical beauty.

INCIDENCE AND AGE OF IDENTIFICATION

How many of the total number of same-sex-attracted teens self-identify as gay and at what age are difficult to determine because investigators use many different ways of assessing sexual identity, including the following:

They admit to themselves that they are gay.
They consider themselves to be gay.
They describe themselves as gay.
They realize they are gay.
They have an identity of being gay.
They label themselves as gay.
They know they really are gay.

Because teens must identify as gay before they can participate in gay-youth research, nearly all studies report that 100 percent of respondents currently have a sexual label. Obviously, based on these data we should not conclude that all teens with same-sex desire label themselves as gay or that a nonidentified same-sex-attracted teen has not accepted his or her sexuality. An Internet study of over 800 young people in which having a sexual label was not a prerequisite for completing the anonymous questionnaire proves this.[17]

Considering only those who attach a sexual label to their personal identity, two trends are noteworthy. First, the age at which individuals first identify as gay appears to be considerably younger among today's generation of young people than among previous cohorts. It has decreased by at least five years (more for females) from those growing up in the 1960s and 1970s. From age twenty-one to sixteen is a large and meaningful decrease: from the end of college or the first years in the workplace to sophomore year in high school, from living out of the family home to living in the home.

A second trend is that sex differences in age of self-identification have largely disappeared. Previously, one could comfortably calculate the average age when males first identified as gay by taking the average age for females and subtracting a year or two. No longer. The average age of self-labeling for a 2000 teen cohort is 16 for females and

15.6 for males.[18] Why this gender equalization? Perhaps the sexual revolution has allowed a greater recognition and identification of a young woman's sexuality than in previous generations.

This revolution has not, however, affected all aspects of sexuality equally. Males and females, at least for the time being, remain at odds in the sequencing of sex and labeling. Traditionally, same-sex contact occurred a year or two prior to a boy's gay identification, while a girl was more likely to have her first same-sex contact *after* identifying as lesbian.[19] This difference was attributed to the greater license to be sexual granted to adolescent boys than girls. If this reason is so, then this difference, too, appears to be fading as girls more frequently question their sexuality and have sex with other girls at earlier ages. The temporal trend also works in the opposite direction. As boys identify as gay at earlier ages, more do so prior to having sex. One general difference, however, remains between girls and boys. Consistent with their heterosexual sisters, same-sex-attracted girls are more influenced in their psychosexual development than boys by interpersonal and situational factors.[20]

Ethnicity can also affect developmental histories, although why this is the case is usually left unaddressed. Although white and African American young men do not differ in age of self-labeling, the latter are less likely to label themselves as gay and are less likely to reveal that they are gay to friends and family. Perhaps being gay is an affront to their ethnic identity in a way not experienced by white young men. Latino young men in the sample self-label and disclose themselves as gay several years before either African American or white young men. Why? Perhaps because of the selective nature of the Latinos who happened to volunteer for the study—femme young men who had been pushed out by their gender nonconformity.[21]

There is nearly always a shorter time span between an adolescent girl's awareness of her sexuality and self-labeling compared to an adolescent boy's. In one study, the average girl took just over three years to move from first awareness to first self-labeling. For the average boy, the figure was five years. This difference between the sexes, like so many others, is decreasing in recent cohorts. Nevertheless, even with regard to today's teenagers, the time lapse between milestones for an individual adolescent can be great or nonexistent—over a decade, or instantaneous.[22]

Despite my own complicity in publicizing these conclusions, I am aware that several problems plague this research.[23] Many studies confuse assessments of sexual identity with sexual orientation, calling it one thing and measuring the other. For interviewers to ask, point blank, "Are you gay?" is too vague. Then, to follow up that question with "When did you know it?" and "What led to it?" further confuses things. Each person to whom they address these questions might take the questions to mean something different—identity, sexual orientation, or sexual behavior. Under these circumstances, both interpreting the data and making comparisons across individuals, groups, and studies are difficult, if not impossible.

Also problematic is the fact that many samples are severely unrepresentative. One might assume that early research based on hustlers and runaways is more biased than recent research based on "out" high school students. But is it? Both groups are likely to identify as gay at the same age. Yet another problem is that some early studies included a wide age range of participants: from eighteen to sixty years of age was not unusual. Thus, multiple cohorts may exist within any one study, and these are seldom distinguished.

The significance of this fact is frequently underestimated, a point generally lost in media reports of young people's sexually identifying themselves at younger ages. If, for example, a contemporary sample is composed of individuals younger than twenty-five, then their age of self-identifying is almost certain to be noticeably younger than earlier studies that included groups of adults eighteen to sixty years of age. The former does not include those within the cohort who won't identify until an age older than twenty-five, while the latter does include these individuals. If all these postadolescent identifications were added to the total of the contemporary study, the average age would likely increase significantly.

Even less is known about the significance or evaluation of self-labeling. Perhaps because nearly every sexual identity model contains some version of "identity pride" following "identity acceptance," researchers generally interpret this milestone as the need to "feel positive" about one's sexuality.

Feeling Good about Being Gay

Perhaps surprising to researchers who emphasize the suicidality, depression, victimization, prostitution, and substance abuse of gay youth,[24] gay teenagers generally feel good about their same-sex sexuality. It might take a few years; maybe even a lifetime. Or it might be instantaneous or exist prior to the adoption of a sexual identity.

In one study, young adults reported feeling good about their sexuality within two years after adopting a gay identity.[25] These findings might strike some as rather surprising, especially because the young people in this particular study grew up in the South in the 1980s. Nearly one third felt good the same year they identified as gay or bisexual. One young man, twenty-four-year-old Irwin, felt good about his sexuality four years before he even reported having a gay identity. Two young adults, nineteen-year-old Kimberly and eighteen-year-old Nathan, never reported having a sexual identity but nevertheless felt good about their sexuality. Herein may be the key. If young people in general have positive self-esteem, they are likely to feel good about their sexual identity.

Another interpretation might be that only self-accepting gays volunteer for research studies. Perhaps, but I tend not to think so. My sense is that same-sex-attracted teens accept themselves at about the same pace as do heterosexual teens. Consider the data reported in Table 8.2. Fully three quarters of same-sex-attracted young people feel very good, good, or indifferent about being gay. Less than one in ten do not want to be gay or hate being queer.[26]

Table 8.2   Feelings about being gay

	(1) M & F	(2) M & F	(3) M	(4) F	(5) M	(6) F
Feel very good	24%	32%	16%	22%	63%	66%
Feel good; wish not a big deal	46%	28%	45%	47%	27%	17%
Doesn't make a difference	9%	30%	13%	17%	6%	13%
Prefer being heterosexual	12%		19%	11%		
Do not want to be queer	4%	7%	5%	3%	3%	2%
Hate; do anything to change	2%	3%	2%	1%	2%	1%

Sources: (1), D'Augelli & Grossman, 2001; (2), Hillier et al., 1998; (3) and (4), Kryzan, 1997; (5) and (6), Kryzan, 2000.

Notes: In (2), terms used were "great," "pretty good," "okay," "pretty bad," "very bad"; in (6), comfort with sexual orientation was assessed as "very," "somewhat," "mixed," "uncomfortable," "very uncomfortable."

Of the young people I interviewed, about nine in ten young women and men developed a positive attitude toward their same-sex sexuality, and they did so on average between their eighteenth and nineteenth years. Whether it is easier for one sex or the other to have a positive evaluation is debatable. On the one hand, because same-sex-attracted girls suffer fewer instances of sexual orientation victimization, including verbal harassment, physical abuse, and sexual abuse, and less often fear parental reaction to their same-sex attractions,[27] one might think that they have the advantage. On the other hand, their lives are less often depicted and celebrated in the media

Labels, Labels, Labels

The sexual identity terms adopted by young people reflect values, as one writer put it, "of relationships, of belonging, of difference and diversity. They provide continuous possibilities for invention and reinvention, open processes through which change can happen."[28] Traditionally, the choices to be selected have been clear. You are homosexual or heterosexual or, more recently, you are gay, lesbian, bisexual, or straight.

Over the last several years, however, other labels have crept into the teenage lexicon, especially among young women. Indeed, only a minority of same-sex-attracted women say they are lesbian. Bisexual is more often preferred.[29] When given the opportunity to choose their own identity term—and not just one but as many as they want—Paula Rodríguez Rust discovered that bisexual adults select on average 2.6 terms. Some choose 10 or more. Particularly popular are compound identities, especially bisexual with modifiers (for example, bi-lesbian, bi-queer). This, in the words of Rodríguez Rust, is a method of "bisexualizing a monosexual identity," a means by which her respondents can express their distaste and, at times, loathing of labels and the implied sexual scripts they seemed to dictate. "Bisexual" is the broadest, least defining, and least offensive term.[30]

The following are some of the words and phrases used by women who claimed physical or romantic attractions to other women:[31]

ambisexual
attracted to females
attracted to the person
attracted to a special woman
bi-lesbian
bi-queer
bisexual
bisexual, depends on person
bisexual in lesbian relationship
bisexual transgender
dating/loving a woman
dyke
female-identified bisexual
fluid bisexual
gay
heterosexual
heterosexual, lesbian tendencies

heterosexual-identified bisexual
heterosexual with bisexuality
heterosexual with questions
lesbian
lesbian-identified bisexual
lesbian who has sex with men
not straight
pansensual
pansexual
polyfide
polysexual
questioning
queer
unlabeled

This does not mean that today's same-sex-attracted individuals are forsaking the usual terms of gay, lesbian, and bisexual. It does indicate a greater flexibility (and, might I add, creativity) in sexual labeling. Perhaps of all the traditional terms, bisexuality is most open to reinterpretation because it bridges sexualities.

Bisexuality

The primary dilemma facing bisexuals in terms of fitting them into traditional sexual identity models is that many bisexuals are fluid in their identity. This makes it difficult to view bisexuality as a static termination point of a developmental process of self-discovery. The models are seldom sufficiently flexible to consider bisexuality as anything other than a transitional identity or a state of identity confusion, even though it may actually be a fully integrated identity.[32]

To address this problem, several scholars have proposed stage models specifically for bisexuals. Parallels have also been drawn between bisexual and biracial identity formation. It is thought that both

those who are bisexual and those who are biracial experience comparable stages of questioning/confusion, refusal/suppression, infusion/
exploration, and resolution/acceptance.[33] However, similar to Alfred
Kinsey, most models present bisexuals as half homosexual and half
heterosexual, or somewhere between homosexuality and heterosexuality. Bisexuals disagree, but their perspective is often neglected.

The view of bisexuality as a compromise to the self-concept is elo-
quently stated by Gil Herdt and Andy Boxer in one of the earliest
studies of gay youth:

> For the vast majority of the Horizons group, bisexuality is a pur-
> chase on time, both social and developmental time . . . The bi-
> sexual, in sum, is a chameleon, an embryonic being akin to the
> trickster of American Indian folklore, full of possibilities to be
> all and everything, but elusive to others and perplexing for the
> self that would fix a steady gaze on its own life.

By the time such individuals reach age twenty-one, Herdt and Boxer
conclude, most "will be in largely exclusive same-sex relations."
Later, however, they switch and reject this notion, having determined
that bisexuality is "increasingly [being] accepted by a generation of
younger people who resist identification with the main categories of
sexual identity."[34]

Margaret Rosario and her colleagues supply empirical support for
the transitional view of bisexuality, at least for those who eventually
identify as gay.[35] At the time of their interviews, nearly two thirds of
the young gay and lesbian respondents regarded themselves in the
past as bisexual, if even for a brief time. However, I find these data
instead to be evidence for the fluidity of sexual identity during the
adolescent years rather than evidence of the instability of a bisexual identity. After all (though this fact is largely ignored by Rosario
and her colleagues), nearly two thirds of the self-identified bisexuals
thought in the past that they might be lesbian or gay. Yet few believe

Table 8.3 Types of bisexuality

Type	Definition
Situational	Heterosexuals engage in same-sex behavior given extenuating restrictive circumstances (e.g., prison).
Chic	Heterosexuals engage in same-sex behavior for social acceptance (e.g., swingers group).
Transitional	Individuals use bisexuality as a bridge to change from one identity to another.
Historic	Sexual histories include behaviors/fantasies contrary to current identification.
Sequential	Consecutive relationships with different genders over time such that at any one point individuals are involved with only one gender.
Concurrent	Individuals maintain relationships with both genders at the same time.
Experimental	Individuals try out relationships with more than one gender as a test for which gender most appeals to them.
Technical	Individuals have sex with both genders but prefer to be lesbian/gay.
Cop-out	Individuals want the "best of both worlds" without having to commit themselves to a particular partner or lifestyle.

that being gay or lesbian is a transitional identity for bisexuals. In nearly every study conducted to date with adolescents and young adults, a sizable fraction freely selects the term "bisexual" to describe their sexuality. Is this transitional? a cop-out? true? Clearly, we don't know what teens *mean* by bisexual. Table 8.3 summarizes the major types of bisexuality that have been proposed in the literature.

Paula Rodríguez Rust has reviewed over 1,000 articles, books, and chapters on bisexuality. She acknowledges that much of the literature assumes that bisexuals are in transition between their former heterosexual selves and their future gay or lesbian selves. Bisexuals supposedly fear the consequences of identifying as gay. They're either in denial about their "true" identity or are unwilling to place themselves into a socially oppressed group. After all, they can "pass" as straight.

"Despite widespread belief in their nonexistence," notes Rodríguez Rust, bisexuals "are stereotyped as psychologically conflicted, emotionally immature, and sexually promiscuous."[36]

As a result, bisexuals are typically excluded or combined with gays, as if they are the same entity. Despite the limited data, Rodríguez Rust asserts that some things are known.

- Bisexual attractions and behaviors are more common than exclusively same-sex attractions and behaviors, but the prevalence of a bisexual identity is less common than a gay or lesbian one. Rodríguez Rust attributes this to the absence of cultural validation and support for a bisexual identity. Both heterosexuals and gays express disdain for "double agent" bisexuals—reflections of bi-phobia or bi-negativity.
- Young bisexuals tend to recall heteroerotic before homoerotic attractions. Given attractions to both males and females, the more acceptable, less stigmatized heterosexual feelings might well be recalled as earlier and more characteristic.
- Bisexuals (especially women) prefer serial monogamous relationships and are thus seldom sexually involved simultaneously with both sexes or report that they are equally attracted to both sexes. If involved with both, they have a primary sexual partner who receives most of the resources and time.
- With age, bisexuals gravitate toward involvement with one sex only; they are more likely to say they are exclusively gay or heterosexual and less likely to say they are bisexual.
- Both female and male bisexuals tend to enjoy sexual relations with males and romance with females.
- Bisexuals average more same-sex partners than do heterosexuals, fewer same-sex partners than do lesbians and gays, and more opposite-sex partners than do lesbians and gays, but not necessarily fewer opposite-sex partners than do heterosexuals.
- Bisexuals have long-term romantic relationships, but their rela-

tionships tend not to last as long or to be as monogamous as those of heterosexuals or gays and lesbians. Bisexuals are more likely to reject sexual monogamy as a cultural ideal.

- Bisexuals are less likely to maintain a consistent identity and more likely to reach developmental milestones at later ages. With two disbelieving worlds to confront—heterosexism among heterosexuals and gays who distrust the legitimacy of bisexuality—bisexuals tend to have few supportive communities and thus struggle to achieve developmental milestones.

Rodríguez Rust discovered that women are more likely than men to identify as bisexual and to want to use bisexual as a compound term. Nearly three quarters of the nearly 1,000 respondents in her study reported that they are primarily bisexual in their feelings and capacities, but they rarely noted the relevance of this fact to their sexual behavior. Bisexuality, according to Rodríguez Rust, represents these individuals' "perception that they remain *capable* of feelings for and/or sexual contacts with both women and men—not the fact they have had such feelings and experiences."[37] It is the *potential*, the *capacity* to have feelings toward both sexes that is critical. Why limit oneself to a single gender or to a narrow range of relationships? The sex of a potential partner is seldom the "deal breaker" for bisexuals. They rely on other factors as the basis for their sexual attractions, especially personality or physical (nongenital) characteristics. Anna, a twenty-year-old Australian, expressed this when she wrote on an Internet survey, "I am not attracted to people based on their gender, rather I grow attracted to people based on their personality."[38]

A minority of respondents in Rodríguez Rust's study reported that their bisexual identity reflects their actual sexual interactions. Some identify as bisexual merely for political reasons—as a means to resist monosexism. Labeling themselves as bisexual does not imply that they want to have sex or a relationship with both sexes. Rodríguez Rust concludes, "Individuals can feel sexually attracted to people with whom they would never consent to have sex, and they can fantasize romances with people they would not even want to meet."[39]

How does all of this relate to teenagers? The prevailing view appears to be that although adults might be "truly bisexual," adolescents are only giving in to the moment. In some high school circles, bisexuality is seen as superficially chic and transitional, but it can also be a means by which a teen identifies with a community and expresses political solidarity with all nonheterosexuals. By so doing, a teen combats bisexual invisibility, objects to the reification of sexual labels, and reshapes sexual politics. It might also be a teen's *true* sexual identity, a reflection of attractions, desires, and fantasies for both sexes. Bisexuality might also be the label that best captures a sense of fluidity, a flexible identity that affords greater freedom of expression, potential, openness, and a breaking of boundaries.

Though all of this is true of bisexuality, contemporary teens are also increasingly saying that labeling oneself bisexual is itself limiting and constraining. Among the young women I interviewed, for example, objections to the term "bisexual" centered on four reasons:

1. It causes conflict within the women's community because lesbians do not like it. They think or believe that it reinforces male patriarchy and gives bisexual women access to heterosexual privilege.
2. It emphasizes only the sexual in identity.
3. People seem to believe that it means that one is attracted to each gender equally or that one has both a male and a female lover. To say one is "bisexual" means having equal attractions.
4. The term seems to imply confusion about one's sexuality.

Doing her best to help me understand her complex perspective, one college student reflected several of these concerns:

I am honestly bisexual in my attractions if you mean do I have attractions for both sexes. But I try to lean way over on the female spectrum because I don't think people generally honestly understand bisexuality when I use it. They honestly think I'm confused or I want three-ways or I can't decide or I want lots of sex (well, actually I do!).

I tried to label myself gay but it just didn't feel right because I'm attracted to guys. In high school I was more attracted to guys because I didn't have any sexual experiences with girls, but now honestly, I'm more attracted to females than males but does that mean I call myself a bi-lesbian? A lesbo-bisexual?[40]

Despite its potential for flexibility, the bisexual label remains one part of a three-part sexual identity system. For some, nothing short of rejecting all sexual labels is suitable.

A Heterosexual Sexual Identity?

Are bisexuals trying to mimic heterosexuals in refusing to use sexuality as a basis for differentiation? All adolescents have a sexual orientation and most are interested in sex, but is it accurate to assume that heterosexuals don't interpret their sexuality as meaning they have a sexual identity? All sexual identity models posit that the homosexuality of same-sex-attracted individuals is their defining characteristic. The necessary corollary is that because of their sexuality, they experience a life course substantially different from that of heterosexuals. An additional, though unstated, assumption is that heterosexuals don't have a sexual identity.

In general, this assumption is ignored. Heterosexuality remains uninterpreted, "unmarked." The guiding notion is that heterosexuality is not a salient or central feature of identity, unlike other characteristics such as race, class, occupation, and religion.[41] As the authors of a rare article on heterosexual identity development note:

Research that addresses the ways that heterosexual individuals perceive their own sexual identity is all but nonexistent. Indeed, some scholars may question the extent to which anything exists that might remotely resemble something called "heterosexual identity development," a point demonstrated in the reality that virtually all literature regarding sexual orientation is situated in volumes designed to address lesbian, gay, and bisexual (LGB) issues.[42]

Heterosexuality is seen as normal. Assuming a different stance regarding heterosexuality is so rare that it is essentially pointless to develop theories of identity around this sexual orientation.[43] Heterosexuals' developing a sense of sexual identity is as rare, even meaningless, as North American white people's claiming a racial identity.

Yet many girls, regardless of sexual orientation, do not consider their sexuality to be sufficiently all-inclusive or all-embracing to base their identity on it.[44] Yes, they have objects of lust and desires of love, but this doesn't imply that they have a sexual identity. Some refuse to have a sexual identity or have, at most, a weak or marginal one. In interviews, heterosexual college women and men reported that they seldom think about their sexual identity. They were unaware of how their sexuality might have affected them or their relationships with others. Only three of the women interviewed questioned their sexuality and their assumed heterosexual sexual identity.[45]

For his dissertation, Loren Frankel investigated these issues among heterosexual and gay college men.[46] On the basis of a free-association "Who Am I" measure, fewer than one in ten heterosexual men self-ascribed a sexual identity term ("straight," "heterosexual"). Only two in ten questioned at some point their heterosexuality. Compared to nonidentifying young men, the 10 percent who gave themselves a label are more likely to have gay relatives and to have questioned (usually during middle adolescence) their assumed heterosexuality. The soul-searching, however, appears more connected to their sexual orientation than to their identity. They wondered about their attraction to males, experienced insecurity about their attraction to females, and questioned their curiosity about sexual experimentation with other males. As further evidence for the low priority given to heterosexuality, the straight men were significantly less likely than gay men in the Frankel study to believe their sexuality affects other domains of their life (career, family relations, hobbies, politics).

These data do not support the idea that heteroeroticism has developmental significance for most heterosexuals. Perhaps some heterosexual young people question their sexuality during adolescence, and perhaps some develop primitive outlines of a sexual identity. The extent to which this is true, however, pales by comparison to the assumed sexual identity development of same-sex-oriented young people.

Indeed, two thirds of same-sex-attracted young men noted their sexual identity on Frankel's "Who Am I" exercise.[47] Not two tenths, but nine tenths of them questioned their sexuality, and at an earlier age (early adolescence). It bears noting that, as is the case with heterosexual men, the questioning that these same-sex-attracted men reported is more about orientation than identity. They were not attracted to females but were attracted to males. What most clearly differentiates them from their straight brothers is that at the time the questions meant something about their sexuality and their choice of social activities and friendships. However, fewer than half of the gay men reported that their career, sports, college classes, and hobbies were affected by their same-sex sexuality. In addition, a substantial number (over one third) of the same-sex-oriented young men did not consider sexuality when describing who they are.

These young men and women are the subjects of the last two chapters. They are becoming the norm; they are the ordinary ones.

9

Resilience and Diversity

Sexual identity models are example number one of the tendency to treat all gay people as the same, as a "separate species." Not only are these models wrong for most individuals with a same-sex orientation, they are also harmful because they keep us from understanding the diverse and ever-changing lives of contemporary teenagers. They foster archaic, male-centric views of gay development.

A number of feminist scholars have raised serious objections to sexual identity models, especially in regard to female development. Lisa Diamond, Anne Peplau, Deborah Tolman, Paula Rodríguez Rust, and Lucia O'Sullivan are redirecting the field in a way that allows us to see sexual and romantic adolescent lives that are positive, resilient, diverse, fluid, and without labels. As a partial corrective to the static quality of existing models, I have proposed a differential developmental trajectories perspective, which I believe is a better framework for both investigating and appreciating the life course of contemporary teenagers.

In this chapter and the next I examine teenagers' lives as they are lived today. It is a world of normative homoeroticism and sexual diversity considerably at variance from what most of us experienced during our adolescence. The liabilities of the predominant, negative perspective toward gay adolescence are too severe. Concentrating instead on the resiliency of young people, the positive aspects of growing up with same-sex attractions, and the diversity that characterizes the world they (and we) live in has to be a better choice.

Distinctively Bad?

Many gay-friendly researchers, professionals, activists, and organizations cite a long litany of ways in which gay teens deviate from their heterosexual brothers and sisters. Perhaps they do this to legitimize the pain of growing up gay, to elicit sympathy for gay youth, or to obtain financial or other resources for prevention and/or intervention programs. The finger-pointing is usually directed at an uncaring mainstream culture; the aim is usually to educate professionals in mainstream institutions (especially schools) about the unique needs of gay teens. These gay "advocates" usually portray young gay people as weak and defenseless in the face of a troubled and violent world. Are there no resilient, strong gay teens who cope, survive, and thrive? If gay adolescents are at high risk for committing or attempting suicide, how similar can they be to heterosexual adolescents? One population is thus found to be "normal" and the other is not. Guess which one is not.

Gay youth's unhealthy abnormality is assumed by some to be the result of an inherent developmental anomaly, perhaps genetic, perhaps prenatal environmental, that makes a person homosexual and will continue to affect his or her behavioral adjustment during adolescence. Others maintain that the very state of being gay elicits increased psychosocial harassment, leading to increased levels of victimization, emotional distress, substance abuse, and mental illness.

A recent review of the empirical literature answers the question "Do LGB people have higher prevalences of mental disorders?" with a resounding "yes." The reason? *Minority stress.* "Stigma, prejudice, and discrimination against gay people create a hostile and stressful social environment that causes mental health problems."[1] Although the author of this study recognizes some of the sampling problems I have mentioned in this book, they don't alter his views. Most telling in the studies he reviews, gays are contrasted with heterosexuals but not among themselves; thus, population variations are ignored, especially between the "out, visible, and early identifiers" and the much larger majority of same-sex-attracted individuals.

I find this very puzzling. If one wants to know about female development, one does not sample only self-identified feminists. If wants to know about African Americans' development, one does not sample only self-identified Afrocentric advocates. If one wants to know about same-sex desires, why sample only gay-identified individuals? Granted, some knowledge is gained, but much is lost.

One could argue, as the reviewer just mentioned chose to do, that the omission is acceptable, indeed, that the findings are conservative, because "people who were more secure and healthy were *overrepresented*" (emphasis added). Without actual data, he speculates that those who do not identify themselves as gay or come forward to participate in research are less well adjusted than those who do. The message? Identifying oneself as gay is a healthy thing to do—or that only healthy individuals are willing to identify themselves as gay.

This notion, however, is contrary to several recent studies. One found that two significant predictors of youth who attempted suicide were disclosure to others of their same-sex status and attendance at support groups.[2] These are the "out, visible, and early identifiers." Another investigation reported that use of drugs was substantially higher among youth who reported having gay sex and identifying as lesbian, gay, or bisexual, in addition to having sexual thoughts/attractions.[3] These are also the "out, visible, and early identifiers." These findings suggest that it is the *nonidentifying* same-sex-attracted teens who are likely to be more healthy.

Indeed, I predict that it is not the existence of same-sex attractions that is a "risk factor" for psychological problems, but the intra-psychic and social pressures that lead a young person (especially at an early age) to identify as lesbian, gay, or bisexual. Further, I suspect that it's not the identity per se that is unhealthy, that leads to suicide or substance abuse, but the personal and social characteristics that coexist with the label, the identity. Identifying as gay during adolescence might be a troubled teenager's attempt to address bad circumstances. Doing so allows him or her to find support, find a distinctiveness, find a community.

Although insufficient data are available to assert with great confidence that teens who identify as gay are less healthy than non–gay-identified teens with same-sex desire, my main objection is to the overarching deficit model. This view leads far too many to search for, and thus unearth, problems among gay adolescents. Indeed, this bias is so entrenched that it causes researchers occasionally to interpret positive findings in the worst possible light. For example, only 3 percent of youth in one study reported feeling really bad or had great difficulty accepting their same-sex attractions. Yet, apparently not believing their own data, the authors note that many youth who reported positive feelings about their sexuality "had experienced a number of difficulties."[4] Success and happiness are neglected. Isolation and confusion are underscored. Concern with negative societal and interpersonal consequences of a stigmatized sexuality are highlighted. It is as though positive gay development can't really happen—there must be a negative underbelly somewhere. Who can be surprised when a review of health-related articles on gay youth published since the 1970s revealed that the most frequent topics have been suicide, HIV/AIDS infection, victimization/violence, sexually transmitted diseases, pregnancy, confidentiality, HIV testing, and sexual abuse.[5] This is not a pretty picture of being young and gay.

This scholarly obsession with the destructive and the injurious can be attributed, as noted in Chapter 1, to two developments. First, early empirical studies and mental health alerts by clinicians, psychiatrists, social workers, and educators set the tone. They decided that gay youth would be perceived as a unique class of individuals in need of clinical services. The equation of "gay youth" with "troubled youth" became so ingrained that any other caricature went undocumented and thus unnoticed. The "not so troubled typical gay teen" remained largely invisible.

A second major development was that early research on the nature of adolescent homoeroticism was derived from the reports of individuals who identified as gay during adolescence. These early identifiers tended to be so sex-atypical in their gender expressions that they were unable to hide their sexuality. They were pulled out of the closet by peers because of their "girlish" or "tomboyish" behavior, or pushed out of the closet by their own internal turmoil, and were thus ideally situated to be harassed by school and neighborhood bullies, to be rejected by parents, to live in dysfunctional families who offered little concomitant hope for support or understanding, to have a mental illness, to abuse substances, to face social isolation. Given this kind of background, claiming a gay identity and participating in gay research were understandable efforts on the part of gay young people to find support, connect with a community, seek cathartic revenge against oppressors, and tell their own side of the story.

So strongly has this image taken hold that even well-meaning parents doubt that being gay is a decent outcome for their child. She'll have a difficult life, thrown out of the military, victimized. He'll be bullied, excluded from jobs, unable to parent.[6] School psychologists, counselors, social workers, and nurses hold similarly negative expectations of their gay students. They overwhelmingly believe that gay high school students are at risk for the following problems (the percentage agreeing is given in parentheses):[7]

anxiety, depression, suicide attempts, harassment (90 percent)
low self-esteem (80 percent)
substance abuse (70 percent)

sexual abuse (60 percent)

dropping out/truancy, eating disorders, unprotected sex (50 percent)

low academic achievement (40 percent)

A new approach, a new attitude is required to reverse the "clin-icalization" of gay youth. Nearly thirty years after major mental health organizations removed homosexuality from their list of mental disorders as laid out in the *Diagnostic and Statistical Manual of Mental Disorders*, gay teens continue to be treated by professionals as pariahs. Just as gay adults were being freed from the rolls of the disabled and dysfunctional, gay young people filled their place. Scientists and clinicians alike have actually *repathologized* homosexuality by portraying gay teenagers as exceptionally vulnerable individuals leading high-risk lives.

Distinctively Good?

An alternative perspective is possible: *resiliency*. The acknowledgment that many teens with same-sex desire are healthy, life-affirming individuals capable of effectively coping with the stresses of life, including those related to their sexuality.[8] Describing these young people as resilient acknowledges the developmental assets they've accumulated over their life course—abilities, traits, and ways of circumventing adversity and health-damaging behaviors and promoting outcomes that are better than one would expect given the amount of risk factors they have.[9] The risk factors have been well documented; the protective factors, which can be innate or environmental (including good schools and families), have not.

As early as the late 1980s, investigators were being warned about the negative imbalance in their research. Absent were data on "features associated with the capacity to remain resilient when confronted by adverse life circumstances."[10] Tony D'Augelli reminded fellow educators in the 1990s to appreciate the exceptionality of gay students and to "encourage them to plan their own development in an active, assertive manner."[11] Few listened. That is not to say, however, that healthy profiles of same-sex-attracted teens don't exist.

The easiest way to demonstrate resiliency is to take a good look at the "doom and gloom" investigations—demonstrate the nonvalidity of data supporting the ill-health of nonheterosexual populations. This is easy to do because the studies are so methodologically flawed that one has to wonder why they were ever believed in the first place, except if they served some agenda.

A simple example will suffice. Reviewers of the literature on gay youths' suicidality report a wide range of prevalence rates for suicide attempts. Most consider 30 percent to be a fair average.[12] Two studies, often ignored in this calculation, relied on sexual *orientation* measures rather than on sexual *identification;* the two found a considerably lower rate—in the 10 percent range.[13] Although the overwhelming consensus is that gay young people are highly and disproportionately at risk for attempting suicide, few researchers note that the majority—an average of 70 percent but possibly as high as 90 percent—do *not* attempt suicide. Given the documented levels of intimidation and harassment young gay people receive, the fact that the vast majority of them do not attempt suicide is noteworthy; it suggests that these teenagers have exceptional, but unacknowledged, coping skills and resiliency.

Several recent studies reflect this kind of alternative approach. They reveal the health and adaptability of same-sex-attracted teens. Over 90 percent of the young people in one study reported that they received support from "real life" (non–Internet world) after publicly disclosing their same-sex attractions. This, notes the study's authors, illustrates the teens' ability to develop "complicated and sophisticated procedures for keeping themselves safe if they feel threatened."[14] Similarly, same-sex-attracted teens tend to be smart in selecting those to whom they first disclose their sexuality. Nearly all first disclosures result in positive, and sometimes enthusiastic, responses.[15]

A third study found that, unlike their white sexual-minority peers, black, Asian, and Hispanic students did not experience significantly more negative attitudes, events, expectations, and performance in school than their heterosexual counterparts. The authors suggest that the experience of ethnic prejudice and discrimination "inoculated" youth against the sexual prejudice they received in school settings.[16]

African American young men with same-sex attractions can create an "integrated and positive identity" through their psychological adjustment to a socially stigmatized role. According to one study:

The male adolescent who identifies himself as a homosexual can function appropriately within his heterosexual environment, as demonstrated by the sample of respondents in this study, if he develops an identity that is capable of withstanding the homophobic attitudes he will experience.[17]

This healthy outcome was enhanced, in part, by the young men's careful, modulated approach to "being gay" and to disclosure. Although these adolescents were not generally publicly "out" because of their desire to maintain a heterosexual image, their best friends knew, and they had gay friends. None of the young men had been, nor felt they needed to be, in professional counseling. Few were upset at the thought of being homosexual.

Finally, a nationally based survey reveals that those who have had same-sex partners since age eighteen did not differ from the general population on a number of variables, including happiness, job satisfaction, substance abuse, perceived health, participation in sports, nervous breakdowns, mental health problems, being punched or beaten, suffering trauma, knowing someone who committed suicide, having positive feelings, and having negative feelings.[18] Another review of the literature reports few differences in quality of life based on sexual orientation.[19]

In the real world, removed from professional hand-wringing over whether gay people are mentally ill, the possibility of positive gay development and resiliency is increasingly apparent. Elite-college re-cruiters view gay-identified high school students as an appealing new niche because of these young people's assumed moxie, toughness, and resolve. Coping with the coming-out experience in high school breeds characteristics that colleges want in their students: self-con-fidence, leadership abilities, and cultural awareness. In addition, the experience of being gay has taught young people to question norms and assumptions, a characteristic of leadership and achievement. But recruiters face a unique difficulty: How can they identify gay high schoolers? Always market-savvy, they attend gay pride fairs, events, and marches. They consult with students on key words to convey their gay-positive views. They note GSA attendants. They search for sensitivity to diversity issues among college applicants.[20]

Another real-world example of gay resiliency is found at a popu-lar Web site for teens, www.YoungGayAmerica.com. Neither of the two Web site creators, Benjie Nycum and Mike Glatze, has a PhD in youth development. The site is not supported by academic in-stitutions or funds. Featured interviews ("the data") do not conform to scientific standards. The mission statement includes the goal of "promoting positive self-image and sense of belonging." Benjie and Mike tour North America, interviewing young people with same-sex desires and posting their stories, pictures, and adventures on the site and in their travel exhibit, called "Exuberance!" So, too, www.outproud.org, with its online magazine, *Oasis*, seeks the same goals. And the Matthew Shepard Foundation's coffee-table book of photographs of diverse and happy gay men and women of all ages, sizes, and races celebrates the lives of same-sex-attracted teens.[21]

Scholars can also contribute to the demise of deficiency models by celebrating the remarkable abilities and talents of young people with same-sex attractions. Models of development from an asset-oriented or positive psychology perspective are allowed. It is not yet too late for social scientists to reclaim the study of gay adolescence and assert their place as the proper and rightful scholars for developing knowledge about same-sex-attracted adolescents. The first step is for them to apply appropriate levels of methodological rigor and sophistication in their investigations. The second is to appreciate the diversity of same-sex attractions and individuals.

Diversity

Jonathan Alexander argues that diversity is both the greatest treasure and the biggest hurdle in the field of what has come to be known as queer studies.[22] In the current epoch of greater cultural visibility and political protection, any notion of the singularity of gayness should disappear. Yet the academy and the government continue to allude to gays as a single entity. Gay lobbying and interest groups are just as guilty of this in their quest for political unity. The reality is that gay people are diverse and at times paradoxical in how they identify themselves, in their politics and political strategies, and in the degree to which they assimilate or want to assimilate into mainstream culture

This diversity is openly and at times embarrassingly displayed in gay publications and personal conversations. Pick a topic, and I can assure you that similarity in sex partner preference does not imply unity in politics or life choices. Fracturing one identity from another can "simultaneously give us a sense of who we are and, at the same time, create divisions and dividing lines between people."[23] The question is, can these natural divisions coexist and remain under the same umbrella? Up to now, the answer has been, "Yes, let's try." However, as the diversity that characterizes people with same-sex desire becomes increasingly apparent, the improbability of this group's being a single population with common points of reference has become increasingly obvious.

In studying gay adolescents, several developmental researchers have acknowledged differences among populations. Jim Sears proposes that growing up gay in the South can be a unique experience

Table 9.1   Adam's five "types" of men who have sex with men

Type	Sex	Love
Not gay	Male and female	Female
Bisexual	Male and female	Male and female
Gay, not bisexual	Male and female	Male
Gay	Male	Male
Queer	Male	Male

Source: Adam, 2000.

because of that region's long-standing culture and traditions. Gil Herdt and Andy Boxer note various sequences of engaging in same- and opposite-sex behavior relative to a gay identification. Paula Rodríguez Rust documents that recording average ages does not adequately capture the diversity inherent among bisexuals.[24]

Based on the gender of sex and lover partners, Barry Adam constructed five "types" among men who have sex with men (Table 9.1).[25] Christopher Hewitt also developed a typology of male homosexuality; his is based on the extent, duration, and timing of sexual engagement (Table 9.2).[26]

Not all typologies have been derived just for males. Margaret Schneider bases her four developmental trajectories from the memories of adult women who recalled their adolescence.[27] Her four trajectories may be described as follows:

1. Early awareness and attractions characterized by the phrase "always knew I was lesbian/bisexual."
2. Heterosexual during adolescence, becoming a lesbian in midlife, usually after falling in love with a woman.
3. Adolescent confusion, turmoil, and considerable vacillation in attractions, with some adopting a bisexual label.
4. Feelings of never fitting in, deferring sexuality during adolescence because of a lack of interest in sexuality in general.

Table 9.2 Hewitt's typology of homosexuality

Type	Self-identity	Social disclosure	Age/marital status	Homosexual behavior	Heterosexual behavior
Open preferential	Gay or bisexual	Open to all	Unmarried	Frequent	Very rare
Repressed preferential	Claims heterosexual	Closeted	Often married	Intermittent and infrequent	Moderate
Bisexual	Gay or bisexual	Varies	Often married	Frequent	Frequent
Experimental	Uncertain	Varies	Young unmarried	Short duration	Infrequent
Situational	Heterosexual	Hidden	Middle-age unmarried	Intermittent	Infrequent

Source: Hewitt, 1998.

Schneider speculates that the essential conditions that activate particular trajectories vary depending on ethnicity, class, temperament, and any other way in which humans distinguish themselves. Yet each developmental milestone has a unique meaning and importance for a particular individual. As Schneider notes, "When participants identify their own milestones, they name a variety of events and cognitions that have far more variation than is reflected in existing models and the meaning ascribed to some of the milestones run counter to conventional wisdom."[28]

Positive, Resilient, Diverse

If one looks carefully at the lives of same-sex-attracted young people, one can't help being impressed by their power and the skill with which they manage to dodge stereotypic characterizations. Scientific attempts to identify what is "normal" or "typical" for adolescents with same-sex desire give us, according to Deborah Tolman and Lisa Diamond, "an impoverished approach." We should discern "not just *whether* factors such as gender, race, ethnicity, and social class are statistically related to specific sexual behaviors, but *how and why* these factors bear a meaningful relationship to adolescents' experiences of their sexuality."[29]

Perhaps the most important first step we should take is to break traditional barriers that prohibit a forthright, positive discussion about sexuality with adolescents. Michele Fine has done this in schools by exploring how school policies and sex education programs portray the sexuality of girls differently from that of boys. Deborah Tolman has done this in communities by comparing the qualities of urban and suburban girls' experience of their sexual desires and how they influence these young women's self-perceptions and sexual decision making.[30]

In these discussions, researchers must assume a realistic and positive mind-set, and must set aside preconceived developmental trajectories, such as that a same-sex-attracted teenage girl should have an early and continuous awareness of her same-sex attractions, and that the sexual attractions she feels must be exclusively same-sex. If the researcher does not set aside such preconceptions and the young woman being studied does not share this normative sequence—for example, if she has never experienced feelings of differentness, sex atypicality, and attraction to and fascination with same-sex others (the experiences researchers think are the best childhood predictors of a same-sex orientation)—she may well feel "doubly deviant."[31] Yet her developmental history, according to Lisa Diamond, would not be deviant or unusual.[32]

Such a young woman could join many other contemporary adolescents with same-sex attractions who are constructing sexual and romantic lives that are not only positive and resilient, but also diverse, fluid, and nonnormative. Scholars might be duped by the male bias or developmental preconceptions of previous research, but teens can teach us a great deal about the incredible diversity that makes up their lives.[33]

The harbingers of such an extensive revision of how we see same-sex-attracted lives have been largely young women. Why young women? Paula Rodríguez Rust attributes the greater diversity, flexibility, and internal inconsistency to women's socialization.[34] Adolescent girls are affected four ways by their cultural training:

1. It allows them to be emotionally expressive and intimate in same-sex relations, resulting in greater freedom to explore affectionate feelings for others of their sex.
2. It inhibits them from expressing their sexuality outright, resulting in more discrepancies between feeling and behavior.
3. It teaches them to derive an identity through relationships and to seek sex within that context, resulting in parallel changes in relationships and identities.
4. It increases politicization of nonheterosexual identities, result-

ing in increased discrepancies among sexual identity, feelings, and behavior.

By conventional standards, developmental "inconsistencies" among women are thus created. Rodríguez Rust points out that

[i]f women are less likely than men to treat sexual identity as a unitary reflection of individual essence and more likely to use sexual self-identity to reflect their romantic, social, and political relationships with others as well as their sexual feelings and behaviors, then that which appears to be inconsistency from a masculinist point of view is, in fact, a different form of consistency.[35]

What these young women teach us is that a singular view of the adolescence of the same-sex-attracted teen is misdirected, if not absurd. They teach us that we must become aware of the resilient adolescent, the one who is coping quite nicely with the vicissitudes of life. These adolescents are already present in our lives. We just need to see them, to move beyond our well-intended efforts to portray the injustices and the harmful effects of mainstream cultural forces. Why not learn something about the effective coping abilities of teens that facilitate the negotiation of a healthy life? Given our long-standing preconceptions, it is perhaps not surprising that we fail to anticipate the possibility that teens with same-sex desire can and do lead productive, happy lives. Their power and resiliency to overcome adversity are embedded in their life stories, and it is these accounts that we should attend to.

My aversion to a problem-obsessed orientation toward gay adolescence is not solely based on my desire to rectify bad science. I want young people to disbelieve the exaggerated news bulletins of high gay youth suicide rates we see in both the popular and the gay press. I realize that some young people will continue to subscribe to the "suffering suicide" script because, in part, it reflects their lives.[36] But these unfortunate young people make up a minority of those with same-sex attractions, so we must be careful not to deliver the message that gay youth suicidality is normative. The important question is not whether gay youth are suicidal, but *which* youth are at risk. With this information we can better determine how effective medical and mental health interventions and services can be delivered for this minority of gay teens.

Targeting "gay youth" generically for special programs might very well increase self-destructive behavior rather than promote wellness; it might encourage the very behavior we're seeking to halt. It might also prevent the healthy behavior we hope to advance, such as the acknowledgment of same-sex attractions. It might also provide sustenance to those who argue that young people should not "choose" to be gay because being gay inevitably results in a deadly lifestyle.[37] Those young people who are already troubled are likely the most susceptible to such messages.

Being young, gay, and proud should not be an oxymoron. Young people with same-sex desire are like most adolescents: they are diverse. They indeed can develop into resilient, coping, healthy adults. We can deliver this message without ignoring those who are suffering, sometimes to the point of ending their lives. Many people experience adolescence as a positive and promising period of their lives. There is no reason why those with same-sex attractions should be excluded from this possibility. It is this message that we need to articulate loudly and clearly, and to support in the pages of our professional journals and in the media. Perhaps then teenagers—and others as well—can hear it and believe it.[38]

10

Refusing and Resisting Sexual Identity Labels

For an issue in early 2004, the *Gay and Lesbian Review*, a scholarly journal, asked several senior gay statesmen to reflect on developments during the previous decade. Most sound unhappy with how things are going. Historian Martin Duberman feels compelled to castigate modern gay men and lesbians as wanting to be "just folks," to simply fit in. Rather, writes Duberman, they should be demanding a radical analysis of contemporary culture. "Where is the Gay Liberation Front of 1970 now that we need it?" he asked.[1] Similarly, novelist Sarah Schulman, a founder of the Lesbian Avengers, bemoans the lack of an activist movement among young people.[2] Youth, she says, are being duped into conformity because they believe the media's representation of their lives.

But what if no duping has occurred and it's real? What if young people with same-sex desires are basically content with modern culture and don't desire a critical analysis? What if the media is reflecting, rather than manipulating, the reality of contemporary teens' lives? Maybe real changes in society's politics, laws, and consciousness toward gay people have raised the possibility that sexual orientation is or will soon be irrelevant in all important respects. Writer Michael Hattersley poses these possibilities, and others:

What would it mean to be gay in a world in which the fact that a friend, sibling, aunt, or uncle was gay was about as relevant as her hair color? What are the implications of a world in which GLBT people have become familiar features in the family, the media, literature, and the political scene? Such a scenario would pose a serious challenge to the perpetuation of "gay politics," to say the least; less clear is what would happen to gay and lesbian literature, art, and popular culture.[3]

This is what really frightens the gay movement's senior statesmen. The potential of leading a normal life is not what they want. Their romantic ideal is being transgressive, being the rebel. Hattersley wonders if this attitude is more self-destructive than noble. It can reflect

self-hatred, legal difficulties, mental illness, suicide, family rejection, and thwarted love . . . Who can blame a persecuted and threatened people if they live for the day and seek immediate gratification, or burn to make something new, to survive, to thrive on being different? How would we define ourselves if that were no longer necessary?[4]

In the same special edition, novelist Andrew Holleran also expresses doubts about the overriding significance of being gay. At a dinner with Harvard University students, he wondered, "What was our bond, after all?" Was it appropriate to be segregated at the "gay table?"

Wasn't it better when a student belongs to the common culture? Could identity politics be a mistake? Just what is there in the space between two gay people who meet today? The same old same old, or something new? So why—the question I asked ten years ago—*did* we make so much of our homosexuality?[5]

Today, fewer young people are making so much of their gayness, which is, according to Holleran, "virtually unrecognizable—evaporated, almost, into assimilation and cyberspace."[6] This he finds to be not a source of celebration, but of resignation. But isn't this what gay activists have been supposedly working for during the past four decades—to be treated as equals, as individuals, to have our humanity rather than our sexuality valued? If the analysis in the *Gay and Lesbian Review* is true, we've been successful beyond our wildest dreams!

The Cultural Landscape

Debates about whether and how gay people are similar to or different from heterosexuals have gone on for decades.[7] If gay people are different, then is it a good different or a bad different? Are they creative, witty, and intelligent or promiscuous, immoral, and mentally ill? Should they identify loud and proud or blend in? Should they fight for political rights or seek social acceptance?

It has long been argued whether gay people may, on the one hand, have a distinctive life course that reflects a deep sense of their "queerness," their sense of difference; or, on the other, whether they are basically similar to straight people—that is, whether they look and act like heterosexuals, value marriage and family like heterosexuals, have the same career aspirations, and hold the same mainstream values.[8] A differential developmental trajectories perspective allows that *both* notions are true *and* that remarkable diversity characterizes individuals with same-sex desire. They seek to adapt to mainstream culture even as they demand acceptance of their sexuality as normative and as they appreciate the increasingly gay quality of the culture.

This real-world complexity is muted among older commentators. The most vociferous among them take extreme positions. One prime example is the writer and activist Larry Kramer, who rants against accommodating gays who he says are losing themselves in the massive, vanilla-heterosexual culture. In a *Rolling Stone* article, he argues that a concern about the fate of one's people should stand at the very center of a gay person's being. "We are a body of people, a nation of gays, a huge political group capable of exercising power! . . . We are the straight white man's slaves."[9]

As a college student at Yale University, Larry Kramer recalls that he was "a pretty lonely young gay man . . . It has always been my dream that I'd leave what I could to insure that gay kids at Yale today would have a better time than I did." Naively buying into reports of high gay youth suicide, he reasons that through portrayals of the unique developmental experiences endured by gay youth, their suffering can be alleviated. Gay writers should write about gay people's lives, and universities should teach gay history. The goal? The development of a new gay culture. This, Kramer believes, is the way to "begin to escape this plague [suicide] that continues to kill off our children one by one."[10]

Several other older gay writers agree with Kramer. Michelangelo Signorile rails against gay people who embrace political and social conservatism, and he is contemptuous of the "ex-gay," "too gay," and "postgay" movements that have "slithered onto the scene." Those who reject a gay identity are, according to Signorile, conforming to the dominant heterosexual culture in thought, values, looks, lifestyle, and political complacency.[11] Similarly, social critics Michael Bronski and Jeffrey Weeks warn about the perils of blending. Gay sex, they say, is central to being gay, to being different from straights, to forging gay identities.[12]

Nothing could be more foreign to young people today than these senior perspectives. The vast majority of same-sex-attracted teens dismiss these extreme stands. Rather, they simultaneously highlight their commonalities with humanity while challenging, according to D'Emilio, "the dehumanizing stereotypes that weigh heavily on our lives and target us for oppression."[13] The culture of contemporary teenagers easily incorporates its homoerotic members. It's more than being gay-friendly. It's being gay-blind.

James Getzlaff, star of the 2003 television reality show *Boy Meets Boy*, reacts negatively to being tricked by the show's producers, who secretly included straight men pretending to be gay among the mix of fifteen men from whom he could choose a date. He says, "The last thing we need is to have anyone think of us as a joke or to make fun of us just for entertainment. We try so hard to put out a positive image as just normal people, looking for the same stuff everyone else is, and that's what I was hoping for."[14]

Those responsible for the show contend that they support accommodation goals. Douglas Ross, the executive producer and codirector of *Boy Meets Boy*, says that he wants his "truly groundbreaking television" show to appeal to a broad audience. "We anticipate a lot of both gay and straight viewers will have their assumptions challenged about what it means to be gay and what it means to be straight."[15] By exploring the sociology of male stereotypes, Ross says, the show promotes accommodation:

> [W]hat are we to make of these straight men who were willing to pretend they were gay and were comfortable enough with themselves to admit that they don't embody the perfect macho image of "straight"? It certainly suggests an evolution in the consciousness of some straight men; and it seems to me that the program did have the effect of shattering stereotypes for both gay and straight viewers.[16]

So, too, other recent television shows with a youthful audience ease the separation between gay and straight. Some examples:

Queer Eye for the Straight Guy, according to reviewer Art Cohen, is "about straight men seeking the advice of gay men, laughing with them, and wanting to be more like them."[17]

The L Word presents women-loving women as totally enviable. The lesbians portrayed on this show tend to be beautiful, ambitious, modern women who have no work problems, zero percent body fat, blindingly white teeth, and constant sex, living in a glowing and delectable world.[18]

In a recent episode of *South Park*, Butters confesses, "Now you know my terrible secret!" Stan reassures him, "You're gay? I don't mind you're gay. That's okay with me."

On the television show *Oliver Beene*, actor Taylor Emerson portrays Michael, an eleven-year-old whose interests and mannerisms quite clearly characterize him as a future gay man (confirmed by a flash forward).[19]

MTV's Chicago edition of *Real World* features Aneesa and Chris, two attractive participants who are not straight.[20]

On *Boston Public*, bisexual high school senior Jeremy Peters is reported to have had anal sex with another guy.[21]

This perspective is readily apparent in many other aspects of young people's lives, all of which tell of a dramatic cultural shift. In sports, high school honor student and varsity athlete Jason Fasi asks his teammates for signatures in support of forming a Gay-Straight Alliance group at Mission Viejo, California. They sign. No one beats him up, no one shies away from dressing next to him, and no one heckles him.[22] Two Ohio high school heterosexual runners wear flashy rainbow socks, symbolic of gay pride, during a state track meet to show support for their two gay teammates.[23]

In the movies, two "straight but spunky" girls decide to make their friendship more complete by testing out a lesbian relationship in *Kissing Jessica Stein*.[24] Young *Harry Potter* actor Sean Biggerstaff receives a ton of fan mail, not all from girls.[25]

A Kaiser Family Foundation and *Seventeen* magazine poll finds that the proportion of thirteen- to nineteen-year-olds who "don't have any problem" with homosexuality more than triples, to 54 percent, during the 1990s.[26] Two Illinois girls are voted the school's "cutest couple" by their fellow high school seniors.[27] Lesbian nineteen-year-old twin sisters, Tegan and Sara Quin, tour North America performing songs from their new musical CD that promote tolerance and acceptance.[28]

Perhaps young people didn't notice that the newest version of the popular computer game, The Sims, has gay characters.[29] Or that the first baby born in the nation's capital in 2003 has two mothers, Helen Rubin and Joanna Bare.[30] This younger generation is amused by the invention of the "metrosexual," but they're surprised that a straight urban male with enough feminine affinities and ambiguity in his sexuality to make him attractive to both sexes creates such a stir.[31]

This shift is reflected in two articles in *Rolling Stone* magazine. Several years ago a feature article, "To Be Young and Gay," recounted the growing number of teenagers who were coming out of the closet and were finding peer and family acceptance. The author, David Lipsky, concludes that gay adolescence is being redefined as a time of angst and struggle *and* as a time of pleasure, acceptance, and limitless possibilities.[32] Three years later in the same magazine, author Jay Dixit reports further refinement. Same-sex-attracted students at Kramer's university no longer feel that "being gay" is a primary aspect of their identity. Gayness has been "backgrounded," as indicated by the following quotes from Yale students Dixit talked with:

A lot of people don't feel the need to foreground that part of their identity. Most gay people spend the majority of their time outside of strictly gay situations.

There's a prevailing attitude of, because I'm gay, it doesn't mean that's my life. I'm not a "gay person," I'm a person who happens to be gay.

It makes it possible to just go about your daily life, rather than having to sit around reminding yourself that you're gay all the time, fighting for all these causes.[33]

Rather than obsessing over their sexuality, these young adults are occupied with typical college pursuits, including sports, fraternities, and careers. One student observes that the "new gay Yalie dresses, talks, and acts no differently than his straight peers." The sex scene is similar to that of straights, with lots of hookups and few long-term romantic relationships. Few assert a gay identity or define themselves in relation to straight culture:

No one really cares or objects to you if you're gay. In fact, making a big deal about being gay is seen as distasteful. The unwritten rule is, you can do whatever you want as long as you don't act like you're part of an embittered minority.

It's sort of avoiding the "I'm here, I'm queer, and I'm pissed off" attitude, because that just turns everybody else off, especially because it's so unnecessary . . . many gay students actually shun activism.

This is going to sound really terrible, but in order to improve their sex lives on campus, people actually try to avoid being labeled as activists. People who are out on the front lines are almost viewed as unpopular in a certain way. I'm not going to use the word stigma, because that's too harsh—but there is a sense of that.[34]

Perhaps these "new gay" or "postgay" students would agree with novelist Armistead Maupin, author of the *Tales of the City* series, who believes that "the only way to lift the stigma of homosexuality is to be matter-of-fact about it." His stories are for everyone and about everyone, regardless of sexual status. Some characters are gay and others aren't. The goal is to normalize the existence of same-sex-attracted people. When asked why he writes about heterosexuals in San Francisco, Maupin refutes the notion that he is "shunning my identity. I want to be myself in the world at large, and that's a far more radical act than confining yourself to a single audience." He claims not to be a gay writer, but a writer who is gay.[35]

Contemporary same-sex-attracted teens essentially agree with the Yalies and Maupin, and not with Kramer and Signorile. Writer bell hooks reminds us, however, of the difficulties faced by marginalized group members if they disagree with the "official position" of their group, such as Kramer and Signorile represent. Is there room for dissent? Although older gay adults may feel pressure to conform to group norms, and this may result in self-censorship and fear that their "minority dissent" will undermine group solidarity, younger people shrug off such pressure. Let the old, professional gays be eccentric, outrageous, and radical, think these members of the younger generation. The oldsters have already lost. Young people have little interest in subverting American civilization. It's the humanity of individuals with same-sex attractions that has won the hearts and minds of middle America.[36] Besides, young people never joined up to be members of a marginalized gay group in the first place.

Why Haven't Teens Signed Up?

What has caused this radical generational shift—from "gay and proud" to "adolescent and proud"? How prevalent is the transformation? What is the difference between same-sex-oriented adolescents who question and identify from those who don't—or between heterosexual adolescents who question and identify as straight from those who don't? What are the factors that determine this? Is it personal experiences? Strength of libido? Does gender matter? How about cohort? How may we best understand the extent to which this indifference to being gay is a healthy outcome? Should teens be encouraged to identify as gay?

I'd like to answer these questions, but I can't. From the information we do have, the information presented in this book, I do know several things. First, adolescents, regardless of sexual orientation, vary in the degree to which sexuality is a core component of their identity. But what makes an individual's sexuality more or less central is baffling. Perhaps it is the degree to which an adolescent feels sexually distinct from the mainstream. A butch girl might centralize a sexual identity because she has encountered unbearable teasing for her supposed lesbianism. Or perhaps the strength of an adolescent's sex drive determines the significance of sexuality for personal identity. An early or particularly significant erotic experience or infatuation might influence the potency of sexual identity. Perhaps it depends on whether the adolescent lives in a home or a community or a time in which sexuality is robust and omnipresent. Maybe the young person has a lesbian aunt or a gay uncle, or other siblings have identified as gay, or friends have come out, and that has influenced the person's degree of gay identity.

Second, adolescents with same-sex desire are not the only ones to question their sexuality, to explore what their sexuality means for their identity. Nor do all adolescents question their sexuality or seek to establish a sexual identity. Sexual orientation per se is not a factor, except to the degree that the individual and the society at large choose to make it one—and this has often been the case, for obvious reasons, given the assumption of universal heterosexuality. Moreover, when we talk only with those for whom sexuality *is* an important and influential aspect of who they are, those who are doing least well with their sexuality, we won't wind up with an accurate picture. Of course these individuals would make much of their sexual identity.

Third, though it is true that an individual's "unorthodox" sexuality may, for reasons alluded to above, result in that person's focusing more on sexual identity than a heterosexual person might, it does not necessarily follow that the full extent of a person's behaviors, perceptions, cognitions, and social interactions is influenced by that sexuality. *Maybe* young gay men as a group are more drawn than straight men to occupations such as interior decorator and flight attendant and are less interested in occupations, such as auto mechanics and athletics. *Maybe* young gay women are more drawn to carpentry and auto mechanics and are less interested in becoming a beauty consultant or fashion model than their straight sisters. The fact is, relatively few same-sex-attracted adolescents actually pursue (or avoid) these occupations.[37] Sexuality can be an important factor in determining career choice, but only for a few. Physical and mental assets, personality, family pressure, and social opportunities are of far greater significance in career choice—for adolescents of all sexual persuasions.

Fourth, despite the speculations of some clinicians, the idea that it is healthy for an adolescent to identify with a sexuality has not been proved. Clinicians are fond of assuming that not adopting a label is unhealthy, that it may be an indication of possible psychological problems.[38] An individual's reluctance to embrace a sexual identity, they say, suggests that the person is in denial, afraid to confront his or her sexual reality. Yet how do we square this view with the overwhelming evidence—produced by these same clinicians—of alarmingly high levels of depression, substance abuse, dangerous sexual activities, and suicidality among those young people who self-identify as gay?[39] Is it possible that self-identifying gay youth are more unhealthy than nonidentified same-sex-attracted young adults?

I believe this is entirely possible. Some gay teens come out "loud and proud" as an act of self-affirmation, and some nonidentified same-sex-attracted young people are in hiding for self-destructive reasons. But it is also true that some declare their sexuality as a cry for help from horrific circumstances and that others are psychologically healthy because they have bases for self-definition other than sexuality that are more developmentally appropriate.

Is it possible that our advice to same-sex-attracted young people has been wrong, and that perhaps we should be encouraging them *not* to identify as gay? Right-wing politicians and ministers advocate this position—but they want more. They want adolescents to *give up* their same-sex sexuality. In this they are naive, because giving up one's sexuality is impossible to do.

As millions of teens are demonstrating, it's possible not to identify oneself sexually and still embrace one's sexuality. The inclination to shun "being gay" can be an adaptive strategy for emotional survival during hostile times and in dangerous environments. Or not identifying can be indicative of a self-loving and wise adolescent. Or perhaps the motivation to self-identify or not has little to do with one's mental health. Gay identity can be indicative of both good and bad mental health.

In these matters, teens with same-sex desire might well mimic heterosexual teens. The fact is, it's a completely individual matter. For Alex, it's his core; sexual identity defines his personal identity. Alex lives in Chicago's Boys Town, is majoring in gay studies with the intent of becoming an attorney who adjudicates same-sex discrimination cases, and writes angry letters to the national gay magazine *The Advocate* because their cover features hot *straight* actors. By attending the Chicago-based youth group Horizons, Alex discovered as a fifteen-year-old "what I needed for myself, that there were other gay people and that gay was not just a phase and that there were older role models." Gay Pride marches, radio interviews, statements to the press—Alex describes himself as a "professional faggot. I'm as queer as they get and proud of it."[40]

In contrast to Alex, Jen tells me that her sexual identity is simply one facet of her core identity and that it has little to do with other aspects of her life. She occasionally attends a meeting of her high school's Gay-Straight Alliance to demonstrate her support for sexual diversity. Only within the last year has she revisited her sexuality.

> Just recently I've put some attention to it. Haven't before because school was occupying my time. Just not enough time because I have a boyfriend. This past summer he was out of the country and I had lots of time and one day I noticed I had undiagnosed strong feelings—I was crying all the time.
>
> This hasn't been easy because I was the first person lots of people told. As a straight ally, I went to Pride Festivals several times, wore supportive ally buttons, but did not attribute anything to myself.[41]

Jen is considering double-dating Lisa with two gay male friends at her high school prom. She prefers not to be so out, however, if it would injure her college applications.

Thomas's sexual identity went unrecognized until he was in college. Then he developed a chaotic, passionate relationship with his roommate.

I wanted desperately to be straight, and the label implied some level of commitment. I dated females and realized that I was attracted to females and so I thought of myself as straight. I sort of let all of this go for awhile and then in the early months of my sophomore year I realized that my feelings for guys must mean something, and it must mean that I'm bisexual. Or maybe what I was, was just sexual.

I've lived with it as if it were a part of me but not that it was real important . . . I don't want to go out and just have sex, but I want to find emotional attractiveness with males like I have with females. Now I know that I prefer males, though I'm probably more bi than most gays.[42]

At the time of the interview, Thomas told me he is engaged and that he plans to marry a woman because it offers what he most wants—an emotional, intimate relationship.

For Sheena, sexual identity is not what she's into—although she loves questioning and thinking about her sexual attractions. When asked she'll say, "I guess I'm heterosexual with lesbian tendencies!" She continues,

If given the right situation and if given a chance, I'd definitely try it, the physical part that is. Friendships with women are so intense, co-dependent-like. I recognized this last week. Always before I had looked the other way, but now I'm willing to consider.

This year has really opened me up, sexually speaking. My best friend came out to me as heterosexual with lesbian tendencies. We were at a party and wasted and she wanted me to French kiss her on the mouth so I did and it was so soft. Sober she'd never do it, but I would. I definitely need my quality girl-time!

So what does this mean? I'm equally attracted to males and females. If, like, I come into a room, I see both the beautiful guys and girls. So I guess I'm 50/50. I see particular qualities in women and this attracts me. I'd love to spend the rest of my life with my best friend. I look at girls the way I look at boys. It's not fair that I can't find boys like her![43]

Sheena admits that these issues are interesting, but she finds that they usually fade to insignificance next to more relevant concerns in her life.

Any idea that adolescent same-sex sexuality is all the same, or that it has predetermined developmental trajectories and consequences, is belied by the life narratives of contemporary teenagers. Their sexuality is but one facet of an interactive system that makes up their lives.[44] Any presumption that teens have identical developmental pathways because they share a same-sex sexuality or that their sexuality is equally important to various teens' sense of self is not only implausible, it is a gross misrepresentation of their lives. The notion of there being a single gay identity or lifestyle is, in short, absurd, especially to adolescents.

To overcome our prevailing misperceptions, we must demystify sexuality and see it as a valid developmental topic, not a clinical risk factor. Sexual development should be seen as a legitimate, growth-promoting, and core aspect of what it means to be an adolescent.[45] At the same time, we must understand that the extent to which sexuality defines identity spans from all-important (it is what I am) to a mere biological fact.

Refusing a Label

A recent survey of a Massachusetts high school revealed that over 11 percent of the students ascribed to themselves at least one aspect of homoeroticism. Seldom, however, did they report having sex with someone of the same gender or identifying as gay. Fewer than 3 percent were willing to assume a gay or bisexual label.[46] In a California high school, 6 percent reported that they "know that I am homosexual or bisexual" and an additional 13 percent said that they frequently or sometimes wonder if they are homosexual.[47]

Naming sexuality as a means to stamp a personal and positive understanding to a life narrative is a relatively recent development. Identifying as gay first became prevalent among those who came of age in the 1970s and 1980s.[48] As Gil Herdt and Andy Boxer put it, people who gave themselves such an identification signified "living with their desires, not in hiding and alienation, but out in the public, in the light of social day—leading to adaptation and greater creative fulfillment than they could have imagined at the beginning of the process."[49]

Although some young people today might also get these advantages from identifying as gay, perhaps especially if they live in secluded, conservative regions of the country, many others object to self-labeling. Some find their sexuality to be more fluid than that permitted by constructed models of sexual identity. Some have notions of what a gay person looks like, acts like, and believes—and it's not them. They cannot or do not want to attribute these features to themselves. Some are philosophically opposed to the idea of placing their sexuality into "identity boxes." To them, the mere creation of sexual categories reifies the labels across time and place and exaggerates differences that don't exist.[50] Some young people give themselves an uncommon or unrecognized label (e.g., two-spirit) or one that encompasses multiple identities (e.g., bi-lesbian). Many simply find the labels an annoyance. One young woman told me:

I felt there just was no need for labels, so I didn't tell anyone. But when I was in tenth [grade] I got interested in this other girl and we were in a romantic relationship. Then I began to define myself differently, more definitely, that it was more real. I just thought labeling was silly, but then people began to ask me for a label. To calm them I said bisexual.

I had wanted to be friends with this girl and then I became more and more interested and then a crush developed. This did not change my self-concept . . . What I wanted to say was that I simply was just in a relationship with a woman. People asked because most of my friends were involved in the gay community and most of my friends were lesbian or gay.[51]

In her work with young people, Beatrice Green observes adolescents who engage in same-sex behavior and yet "refuse the politics of sexual identity, arguing that these are the issues of the older generation. They claim the right to love and have sex with whomever and in any way they want." She refers to them as the "new Act Up generation" and speculates that although they might threaten both the gay and the straight establishment, "they may be the future in a post-identity politics society."[52] I agree.

These young people are repudiating the appropriateness and artificiality of dichotomous definitions of sexual identity as they challenge cultural definitions of gay lives. Gay and straight categories may have been fine for their parents, but not for them. Youth culture is permeated by nuance, especially with regard to sexuality. Sexual behavior and sexual orientation flow within various gender expressions and changing definitions of what is gay, bisexual, and straight. If pushed, they might agree to vague terms such as "queer" or "not straight." Their preference is to not call themselves, or their futures, anything at all. They refuse to label themselves because they wish to separate sexual desire from the friction of politics. One person who was interviewed for a popular article on the "polymorphous normal" asserted that sexuality is not about politics but about pleasure and happiness. Another eschewed identity categories because "my experience is continuous. It's not compartmentalized into poetry and sexuality and rational thought. We confuse the map with the territory."[53]

Some of these young people have been called "queer," defined by anthropologist Melinda Kanner as individuals intent on "destabilizing conventional categories, subverting the identities derived from and normalized by heteropatriarchy. Queerness defies binary and fixed categories such as homo-/heterosexual, female/male, even lesbian/gay. Queerness, in both social performance and in lived identities, interrupts both convention and expectations."[54] Most teens, however, do not think of themselves as queer or appreciate the word. They simply reject the potentially life-altering repercussions of such a label.

Their rejection of label designations is motivated by many things—for philosophical reasons, because the labels seem irrelevant and uncharacteristic, in an attempt to avoid homophobia, or because the label is simply felt to be inaccurate. Some may believe that their current attraction or relationship is a "special" one, an aberration that implies little about them or their sexuality. Others fear the consequences of being gay and so remain unlabeled and closeted, perhaps coming out later in their lives. We know little about these nonidentified teens, but we know they exist.

In a 2001 interview, actor and filmmaker Jason Gould was asked about being gay, coming out, and disclosing his sexuality to his famous parents, Barbra Streisand and Elliott Gould. Jason, who recalled having his first "gay impulse" at age eight, says that he has not come out as gay because he has never said to himself, "Oh, I'm gay." He denies living a closeted life or being ashamed of who he is. "I'm pretty comfortable with my sexuality," he says, adding,

You know, the more I understand my own sexuality the more I . . . I mean I don't mind being called gay, because I'm certainly attracted to men. But I also think that it's limiting. I think that within the gay community—and as a member of the gay community—it's limiting for us to stereotype ourselves. Attraction is more complex than the terms gay, straight, and bisexual. And I hope that eventually people will evolve into accepting a broader understanding of attraction.[55]

Gould's refusal to declare a sexual identity is apparently not a function of internalized homophobia or self-hatred or fear. He has declared his sexuality—he is attracted to men; he simply finds the term "gay" an inadequate descriptor of his sexuality.

Jason Gould is not alone. Comedian Rosie O'Donnell doesn't appreciate the adjective "gay" permanently attached to her name. Being attracted to other women, she says, was never a "big deal for me."[56] Sophia of MTV's *Road Rules* downplays her sexuality: "It's not a big deal to me because I don't make it a big deal . . . It's just part of who I am."[57]

The balkanization of sexuality, according to one writer, is especially prevalent among artists, students, cultural explorers, and young women. They prefer an alternative, self-generated identity label or no label at all rather than those typically offered in research investigations.[58] Two of these groups, young women and cultural explorers, in particular have not been well served by standard sexual taxonomies.[59]

YOUNG WOMEN AND FLUIDITY

Inflexible, distinct boundaries rarely apply to young women's sexuality.[60] A young woman's most enjoyable sexual fantasies might be of other women while her most enjoyable sex is with men—or vice versa. Young women are more likely than young men to incorporate partners of both sexes in their behavior and fantasies. When shown explicit sex films, lesbians and heterosexual women do not differ in their subjective and genital arousal to either male-female or female-female sex scenes,[61] and the highest arousal for both groups of women is to heterosexual sex scenes. In their research, Meredith Chivers and her colleagues suggest that women, regardless of sexual orientation, have a "nonspecific" pattern of sexual arousal.[62] That is, although heterosexual college women might say that they prefer heterosexual over female-female and male-male erotica, their actual genital arousal to sex scenes indicates no significant preference of

211

male-female over female-female scenes. They prefer and become more aroused by female-female than male-male sex scenes. By contrast, gay and heterosexual men show a strong preferred-sex ("categorical") pattern. Gay men are more aroused by male-male than male-female scenes, and heterosexual men are more aroused by male-female scenes, although heterosexual men react most strongly to female-female erotica. Perhaps as a result, women are less apt to be stigmatized for engaging in same-sex behavior.[63]

In eighth grade Stephanie and Lolita were best friends. Stephanie recalled that

> Lolita would sleep over a lot and one night she was talking about her boyfriend Juan and talking about sex. I was pretending to know more than I did. We had been very affectionate, like most girlfriends. I asked her how he kissed her, and so she kissed me like her Juan did. This was quite a shocker. From then on we kissed a lot when we got together, and began touching and caressing. To make it "okay," one of us would be the boy. Was penetration with our fingers but never oral sex. She's straight as far as I know.
>
> Never talked about it. I can't tell what Lolita is, but I was the only girl she did anything with. We never said we were lesbians. I kind of knew that it was not right, but it felt okay. Mom caught us in bed and this was a big uproar. We had gotten together every day after school for six to seven months but Mom made that more difficult.

Stephanie's attitude was that her experience with her friend was just a kid experience. Lots of peers were having sex, only with guys, so having sex was not unusual.[64]

Once a young woman recognizes that she's not totally straight, there is little guarantee that she'll declare herself to be lesbian or bisexual. In an attempt to identify "authentic" lesbians, researchers have traditionally relied on what they believe has worked for identifying gay young men: the achievement of developmental milestones. But, as we have seen, such models won't distinguish lesbians who maintain their lesbian identity over time from those who don't. It is more informative to examine patterns of attraction and behavior.[65]

Over the course of eight years, nearly two thirds of the young women Lisa Diamond interviewed changed identity labels at least once, often because "sexual identity categories failed to represent the vast diversity of sexual and romantic feelings they were capable of experiencing for female and male partners under different circumstances."[66] Some of these women expressed their ambivalence by viewing their sexuality as fluid. Love depends on the person, they told her, not the gender of the person.

Those women Diamond studied who relinquished their lesbian or bisexual identity for a heterosexual or an unlabeled status had similar developmental histories. What differed was their *interpretation* of their sexual experiences. The women who would not be labeled described their sexuality as fluid and expressed uncertainty about their future sex lives. Those who changed to a heterosexual label had lower levels of same-sex attractions and behavior throughout the study than did the other women. A heterosexual identification was, for them, a viable solution to the "problem" of their nonexclusive attractions and behavior.

Relinquishing a sexual identity label, however, did not mean that these women relinquished their same-sex sexuality. Their same-sex attractions and behavior were real, not a phase. All maintained that they might identify as lesbian or bisexual in the future. Diamond noted that

[t]hese findings are consistent with the notion that identity relinquishment does not represent a fundamental change in sexual orientation itself, but rather a change in how women interpret and act upon their sexual orientation . . . Nonexclusivity

213

and plasticity in women's attractions and behaviors potentiate multiple transitions in identification and behavior over the life course.[67]

In short, attempts to fit an adolescent girl's "complex, highly contextualized experiences of same-sex and other-sex sexuality into cookie-cutter molds of 'gay,' 'straight,' and (only recently) 'bisexual'" are doomed to failure.[68] The exception of these young women to follow sexual identity models of identity progression simply reflects the complexity of their lives.

CULTURAL EXPLORERS AND ALIEN NOTIONS

A similar disconnect between orthodoxy and life histories is evident for young people in non-U.S. cultures and subcultures within the United States. In reviewing the cross-cultural evidence, Fernando Luiz Cardoso and Dennis Werner conclude, "People vary tremendously in their same-sex behaviors, in their sexual desires, and in the ways they define themselves. Cultures also differ widely in the ways they define and treat these relationships and the people who engage in them."[69] Western definitions of sexuality are viewed as exceedingly rigid. For example, as one writer notes, in some communities "same-sex relationships are defined between individuals and may involve sexuality, eroticism, and very intensive friendships and emotions. Men can therefore hold hands in public or sleep naked in the same bed together." One Iranian remarks that in his culture labels for sexuality are relatively rare.[70]

It is not difficult to find cross-cultural examples of a homoerotic life that are not identified as such. One has been referred to as "Mediterranean homosexuality." In a culture with this type of sexuality, according to Iñaki Tofiño, a gay activist in Catalonia, there is a "large zone of liberty for homoerotic activity between males, but no such thing as a 'homosexual identity' as such." The sexes are often separated during adolescence and young adulthood; homoerotic friendships, alliances, and physical contact are not uncommon. A person's identity (for both men and women) is not usually defined by what one does sexually or who one falls in love with. To do so would be to deny the more legitimate cultural prescriptions for identification based on religion, region, or ethnicity. To "come out as gay" makes little sense in such a culture. To attach a gay persona "in every situation is an alien notion" and can often be problematic when sex is not part of the public discourse.[71]

Tofiño argues that Western notions of a public or private gay identity that one carries from one situation to the next are not necessary for large-scale cultural changes to take place. For example, in Spain few identify as gay; yet sexual orientation is a category that enjoys broad protections in that country's Penal Code, which acknowledges same-sex couples and provides gays with protection against hate crimes.

An example within the United States of how a gay identity has been subverted is described in a recent *New York Times Magazine* article. Author Benoit Denizet-Lewis explores the world of African American young adult men who have sex and romantic relationships with men and who are forging an "exuberant new identity" based not on their sexuality but their skin color and culture.

> Rejecting a gay culture they perceive as white and effeminate, many black men have settled on a new identity, with its own vocabulary and customs and its own name: Down Low . . . [T]he creation of an organized, underground subculture largely made up of black men who otherwise live straight lives is a phenomenon of the last decade . . . Most DL men identify themselves not as gay or bisexual but first and foremost as black. To them, as to many blacks, that equates to being inherently masculine.[72]

A DL identity signifies a virulent rejection of a gay identity associated with "drag queens or sissies." One eighteen-year-old whom Denizet-Lewis spoke with clearly wants this separation. "Gays are the faggots who dress, talk and act like girls," he said. "That's not me." These men acknowledge the sexuality in their lives, but being DL is not perceived as merely another sexual identity label. It is about "being who you are, but keeping your business to yourself."[73] It is a selection of ethnic affinity over sexuality and masculinity over femininity.

The majority of young people of both sexes with same-sex desire resist and refuse to identify as gay. We know little about them because they usually opt out of research, educational programs, and support groups. Their desire is not to stand out "like a semen stain on a blue dress," but to be as boring as the next person, to buy an SUV and to fade into the fabric of American life.[74]

Ordinary Jane, Ordinary Joe

In the previous chapter I discussed the nascent movement underway to change our preoccupation with deficit models to one that acknowledges the resiliency of gay teens. Although I generally applaud this change—a resiliency script is certainly preferable to a suicidal one—I believe it too is ultimately flawed, for it simply substitutes one universal, overwrought characterization for another. The reality is that both at-risk and resilient gay teens are minor players among the symphony of the same-sex attracted. Most are no more or less resilient or healthy than their straight friends. Most remain, well, *ordinary* as they negotiate routine and uneventful lives.

An alternative perspective, one I believe is closer to the truth, is to recognize not only the positive features of being "different from the norm" but also the *ordinariness* of most young people with same-sex desire. Resistance to this notion is stiff, perhaps less from popular culture than from the world of scholarship and academia, which is blinded to the existence of the ordinary because of the biases inherent in typical survey questions. As the previous chapters have made clear, not all adolescents who experience same-sex desire identify as gay or engage in same-sex activities. Not all adolescents who identify as gay have a same-sex orientation or engage in same-sex behavior. Not all adolescents who have sex with their own gender identify as gay or have same-sex attractions. Scholarship that neglects these facts seldom finds "hidden" populations who have one or two of these features but not all three. Or who have all three, but to varying degrees.

If the "nongay majority with homosexual feelings" group of adolescents could be found,[75] what might be discovered is not their exceptionality but their normal adolescent concerns. Lisa Diamond notes that adolescents with same-sex desires ruminate far more about "love and romance than about suicide, hate crimes, or homelessness, and they currently have nowhere to turn with their concerns."[76] Love does not discriminate based on sexual orientation or the object of one's infatuation. Consider the following quotes—first, from Catherine Deneuve:

> But to be in love with a man or a woman, it's the same thing; it has to do with giving and listening and being very open to someone, so it does not make much difference.[77]

And next, from Dennis Quaid:

> We're attracted to whomever we're attracted to. We can't help loving the people we love, and we can't help being attracted to what we're attracted to.[78]

One needn't identify as gay or engage in same-sex behavior to fall in love with another girl or boy. Indeed, most same-sex lovers do not claim a gay identity. The most accurate, albeit not breathtaking, conclusion is that sexual orientation dictates some of the essence of what it means to be alive, but not everything.

Thus, to understand same-sex-oriented teens we must first understand adolescence in general. Too frequently our investigations ignore the vast theoretical and empirical literature on adolescence in favor of methodologically flawed gay research. Conversely, rarely is it suggested that scholarship on gay youth can add to a general understanding of adolescent development.

Consider John Gottman and his colleagues' recent research on same-sex relationships.[79] Placing their investigation within the larger context of research on couples generally, the team found the following:

1. Similar to heterosexual couples, same-sex couples' expressions of contempt, disgust, and defensiveness are associated with a decrease in relationship satisfaction; humor and affection, to high relationship satisfaction.
2. In situations of conflict, same-sex couples are less belligerent, domineering, and tense and display greater concern with equity, humor, affection, and joy than heterosexual couples. Whereas heterosexual couples often display detachment in times of conflict, same-sex couples become more emotionally and mentally involved and engaged.
3. Within the relationship, lesbians are more likely than gay males to overtly display their affection for each other (emotional expressiveness); gay males are more likely to verbally validate each other. These differences are consistent with sex differences among heterosexuals.

In speculating about these differences, Gottman and his team note that same-sex couples are more likely to value equality and to be more positive toward each other. The inherent status differential between men and women in heterosexual relationships, which "breeds hostility, particularly from women, who tend to have less power than men, and who also typically bring up most of the relationship issues," is largely absent in same-sex couples. According to the authors, "Because there are fewer barriers to leaving homosexual compared to heterosexual relationships, homosexual couples may be more careful in the way they accept influence from one another. Thus, we suggest that the process variables by which they resolve conflicts may be the very glue that keeps these relationships stable."[80] In other words, same-sex couples have something to teach heterosexual couples about respect, equity, and stability.

These dual responsibilities of research on same-sex-attracted young people—rooting research hypotheses and interpretations within the larger context of adolescent development and translating results in terms of how they extend knowledge about adolescence in general—are routinely ignored. It is as if no one has ever conducted research on school achievement, peer harassment, self-esteem, romantic relationships, or family relations prior to our particular investigation of these issues with gay youth.

Given these shortcomings, there should be little wonder that gay teens are believed to experience meaningfully different life trajectories from heterosexual teens. To Middle America, gay teens are arrogant aliens from another culture, at the margins of society with multiple body piercings, purple hair, and pointedly non–Abercrombie and Fitch clothing; to gay adults, they are supposed to be the next generation of political activists who will fight for gay rights and against heterosexism, racism, sexism, and classism.

These young people, however, are neither our enlightened heirs nor our prodigal descendants. Sexual diversity is becoming normalized, and the gay-straight divide is becoming blurred. Straight teens are acting, looking, and becoming gayish, and an expansive array of nonstraight teens is becoming visible. These young people are more apt to say things like "Why won't my parents let me go to the concert?" and "If I take chemistry, how will that affect my grade point average?" than "I'm gay, I'm gay, oh my, what am I going to do?"

This is not to deny that some are ridiculed because of their gender expression. Or that they cannot openly date those they love most because same-sex dating in high school is still difficult for most. Or that they feel they must keep something of themselves secret from their parents and friends. But same-sex-attracted teenagers are not the only young people facing these kinds of problems. Disabled kids, above- and below-average-intelligence kids, unattractive kids, overweight kids, and ethnic-minority kids are also ridiculed. Many teens from these groups do not date the person they desire because they feel that the desired person is "unreachable." Many have profound secrets they do not tell their parents or friends, such as those relating to pregnancy, substance use, nontraditional sexual longings, and psychic beliefs. So why should the life experiences of same-sex-attracted teens only be of such singular significance that they are seen as being unable to cope with their problems and incapable of leading happy, productive lives?

We see gay *adults* as being able to lead happy, healthy, and productive lives; they are said not to differ from heterosexuals in psychological adjustment.[81] We could also see young people this way. Same-sex-attracted young people want to join and become involved in the heterosexual world of their fellow teenagers. A previous generation established "gay proms"—first in Detroit and later in Los Angeles—as a means to build support, pride, and social change. Nowadays, the inclination is to have same-sex couples attend *regular* high school proms. This is the far greater revolution. It normalizes same-sex sexuality in a way that was not possible when only separate gay proms welcomed same-sex couples.[82]

Nothing I have stated in this book justifies neglect of gay young people who suffer and entertain thoughts of suicide because of their sexuality. I am willing to believe that this reality *might* have been more characteristic of earlier generations than it is today. But whatever motivation might prompt us to sensationalize the fate of gay teens or represent them as heroic survivors, it's not scientifically valid now, and it was not scientifically valid in years past.

Both the national and the gay press misrepresent most gay teens and deliver a risky message to those wondering if they might be gay.

Consider the following headlines from various publications over the past several years:

Dying to Be a Boy Scout?
Suicidal Tendencies: Is Anguish over Sexual Orientation Causing
　Gay and Lesbian Teens to Kill Themselves?
Gay Youths' Deadly Despair
Robbie's Story: How a Fragile 14-Year-Old Boy Was Crushed in
　His Struggle to Accept Being Gay
"I Couldn't Have Saved Him the Rest of His Life"
Bad Days for Gay Teenagers
The Hidden Plague[83]

Scholarship must rise above such "doom and gloom" caricature and present the larger context of teenagers' lives.

Why is there such profound resistance to the normalization of same-sex-attracted young people? Why is the focus on the outliers rather than the majority? Here are four (bad) reasons:

1. Because the positive and healthy lives of typical contemporary gay teenagers contradict the tumultuous and painful adolescence of gay scholars and policy makers.
2. Because well-adjusted gay teens present problems for those applying for problem-focused research grants and for the need, as one critic put it, to "manufacture victims for the psychology industry."[84]
3. Because otherwise today's teens would not fully appreciate what researchers, educators, mental health professionals, and activists did for them to allow them to live their lives without fear. How can this "gift" be thrown away so cavalierly?
4. Because today's young people are harbingers of a time in which sexual identity will have no importance, thus thrusting past research into the garbage heap of antiquated science,

making it nothing more than a curiosity for historians and anthropologists.

New gay teenagers disdain sexual categories, and they believe, as Michael Bronski writes, "that some of 'us' have more in common with some of 'them' than we have with each other . . . Within all of these identities are some who are as mainstream as can be, and some who march to their own drummer."[85] It might be wise to listen to their voices and appreciate the reasons they reject the notion of being identified by their sexuality. Led by contemporary young women who are trading in the labels "lesbian" and "bisexual" for descriptors that better reflect their reality, new gay teens are simply trying to live within the flux of adolescence.[86] Their lives, as Jeffrey Weeks observes, provide "continuous possibilities for invention and re-invention, open processes through which change can happen."[87] Some assimilate, and some accommodate. Some embrace gayness, and some refuse it. It's just that the old categories of gay and lesbian don't fit anymore.[88]

Banality

The fact is, the lives of most same-sex-attracted teenagers are not exceptional either in their pathology or their resiliency. Rather, they are ordinary. Gay adolescents have the same developmental concerns, assets, and liabilities as heterosexual adolescents. This unnoteworthy banality might well be their greatest asset. It suggests that they are in the forefront of what can be called a postgay era, in which same-sex-attracted individuals can pursue diverse personal and political goals, whether they be a desire to blend into mainstream society or a fight to radically restructure modern discourse about sexuality.

It is my fervent hope that what is being achieved in the real world can be achieved in scholarship. I hope to see the elimination of same-sex sexuality as *a* defining characteristic of adolescents in my lifetime.

If it can be relegated to insignificance, the lives of millions of teens will be dramatically improved.

I give the final word to "Andrew James," a college student who concluded his essay "In Search of Ordinary Joes" with a simple goal: "Raising the profile of banal homosexuals . . . It's not going to be fabulous, it's not going to be cutting edge, but I think it's got to be the next wave of the gay movement."[89]

Notes

1. WHY THE *NEW* GAY TEENAGER?

1. Wloszczna, 2004; Musto, 2004; Catlin, 2004.
2. Savin-Williams, 1998a, in preparation.
3. Savin-Williams, in preparation.
4. Robb, 2004.
5. Marech, 2004.
6. Savin-Williams, 1998a.
7. Savin-Williams, in preparation.
8. Mead, 1970, p. 60.
9. Hamilton College & Zogby International, 2001.
10. Scheufele, 2004.
11. Dowd, 2003.
12. Yang, 1997.
13. Reuters News Service, 2001.
14. *New York Times*, 2003.
15. Zacharek, 2003.
16. Associated Press, 2003a.
17. *USA Today*, 2003.
18. Sharp, 2003.
19. Quoted in Associated Press, 2003b.
20. Zernike, 2003.

21. Quoted in Associated Press, 2003c.
22. Bronski, 1998.
23. Cohler & Galatzer-Levy, 2000.
24. Lewin, 2004, p. 5.
25. Krauss, 2003, p. 1.
26. Brown, 2002; Sutton et al., 2002; Ward & Rivadeneyra, 1999.
27. Uribe & Harbeck, 1991.
28. Griffin, Lee, Waugh, & Beyer, 2004; Holmes & Cahill, 2004.
29. Herdt et al., 2002; S. T. Russell, personal communication, October 8, 2003.
30. Diamond, 2000a; A. M. L. Pattatucci, personal communication, June 25, 1995.
31. Lippa, 2000.
32. D'Emilio, 2002.

2. WHO'S GAY?

1. Savin-Williams & Ream, 2003b.
2. McWhirter, Sanders, & Reinisch, 1990.
3. Kinsey, Pomeroy, & Martin, 1948.
4. Shively & DeCecco, 1977.
5. Klein, Sepekoff, & Wolf, 1985.
6. Sell, 1996, 1997; Gonsiorek, Sell, & Weinrich, 1995.
7. Coleman, 1990.
8. Friedman et al., 2004.
9. Chung & Katayama, 1996.
10. Horowitz, Weis, & Laflin, 2001.
11. Lock & Steiner, 1999b.
12. Sandfort, 1997, p. 261.
13. Cohen, 1999; Ellis, 1996a, 1996b.
14. Zucker, 2003.
15. Maccoby, 1998, p. 191.
16. Garofalo et al., 1999; Remafedi et al., 1992.
17. Savin-Williams, 1998a.
18. Bell, Weinberg, & Hammersmith, 1981.
19. Cohen, 1999, 2002.
20. D'Augelli & Hershberger, 1993.
21. For example, D'Augelli & Hershberger, 1993.
22. Saewyc et al., 1998; Remafedi et al., 1992; Garofalo et al., 1999, respectively.

23. Upchurch, 2002.
24. Savin-Williams & Diamond, 2004.
25. Peplau & Garnets, 2000; Rodríguez Rust, 2000; Rose, 2000; Rothblum, 2000.
26. Mustanski, 2003.
27. Carpenter, 2001.
28. Mustanski, 2003; Sanders & Reinisch, 1999; Bogaert & Fisher, 1995.
29. Schwarz, 1999.
30. Fine, 1988; Thompson, 1995; Tolman, 2002; Tolman & Diamond, 2001.
31. Savin-Williams & Diamond, 2004.
32. Diamond, 2003c; Weinberg, Williams, & Pryor, 1994.
33. Battle, 1998.
34. Marech, 2004.
35. Savin-Williams & Diamond, 2000.
36. Ibid.
37. Data provided in Diamond, 1998, 2000b, 2003a; Savin-Williams, 2001c; Savin-Williams & Diamond, 1999, 2000.
38. Laumann et al., 1994, p. 283.
39. Sandfort, 1997.
40. Sell, Wells, & Wypij, 1995; Gangestad, Bailey, & Martin, 2000; Sandfort, 1997.
41. Kinsey, Pomeroy, & Martin, 1948; Kinsey et al., 1953.
42. Diamond, 1993, p. 306.
43. Halpern et al., 1993; Garofalo et al., 1999; Faulkner & Cranston, 1998.
44. Remafedi et al., 1992.
45. DuRant, Krowchuk, & Sinal, 1998.
46. Laumann et al., 1994.
47. Gagnon & Simon, 1973.
48. Copas et al., 2002; Papadopoulos, Stamboulides, & Triantafillou, 2000.
49. Sell, Wells, & Wypij, 1995.
50. Garofalo et al., 1999; Remafedi et al., 1992; Laumann et al., 1994; Sell, Wells, & Wypij, 1995; Gangestad, Bailey, & Martin, 2000.
51. Diamond, 2000b, 2003a.
52. L. M. Diamond, personal communication, March 12, 2004.
53. Laumann et al., 1994.
54. Remafedi et al., 1992.
55. Ibid.
56. Savin-Williams & Ream, in preparation–a.
57. Lippa, 2000.

58. Lock & Steiner, 1999a.
59. Rodríguez Rust, 2001.
60. Remafedi et al., 1992.
61. L. M. Diamond, personal communication, March 12, 2004.
62. DuRant, Krowchuk, & Sinal, 1998.
63. Savin-Williams, 1998a.
64. Diamond, 2000b; 2003a.
65. Diamond, 1998.
66. Carballo-Diéguez, 1997; Carrier, 1995; Manalansan, 1996; Savin-Williams, 1996.
67. McConaghy, 1999, pp. 296, 302.

3. IN THE BEGINNING . . . WAS GAY YOUTH

1. Foucault, 1978.
2. D'Emilio & Freedman, 1988; Diamond, 2000a; Faderman, 1981; Smith-Rosenberg, 1985.
3. Faderman, 1977, p. 214.
4. Bullough & Bullough, 1980, p. 123.
5. Tannahill, 1980.
6. Williams, 1986, 1996.
7. Herdt, 1987.
8. Wheatcroft, 1999.
9. Sullivan, 1953, p. 256.
10. Ruoff, 2001.
11. Hall & Simmons, 2001.
12. Roesler & Deisher, 1972, p. 1023.
13. Remafedi, 1987a; 1987b, p. 336.
14. Martin & Hetrick, 1988, p. 172.
15. Rotheram-Borus et al., 1992; 1995, p. 77.
16. Ryan, 2000.
17. Coleman, 1981–1982; Jones, 1978; Malyon, 1981; Martin, 1982; Remafedi, 1985; Tartagni, 1978.
18. Malyon, 1981, p. 321.
19. Coleman, 1981–1982, p. 42.
20. I had taught my first course on the developmental aspects of homosexuality two years earlier and collected data on gay youth three years earlier (Savin-Williams, 1990).
21. Savin-Williams, 1994, p. 262; see also Muehrer, 1995, p. 75.

22. Ryan, 2000.

23. *Journal of Adolescent Health Care*, 9(2), 1988; *Journal of Homosexuality*, 17(1–4), 1989.

24. *High School Journal*, 77 (1994), followed years later by *Journal of Adolescence*, 24(1) in 2001.

25. Savin-Williams, 1998b.

26. Uribe & Harbeck, 1991; Schneider, 1989.

27. DuRant, Krowchuk, and Sinal, 1998; Faulkner & Cranston, 1998; Garofalo et al., 1998, 1999; Remafedi et al., 1998.

28. Sandfort, 1997.

29. Hedblom & Hartman, 1980.

30. Savin-Williams, 2001a; Savin-Williams & Ream, 2003b.

31. The first such survey was begun in 1983 (Savin-Williams, 1990); see also D'Augelli, 1991a; Herdt, 1989; Herdt & Boxer, 1993.

32. Sandfort, 1997, p. 265.

33. Finn, 2004.

34. Wiederman, 1999.

35. Boxer & Cohler, 1989, p. 321, 319; see also Savin-Williams, 1990.

36. Savin-Williams, 1990.

37. Edwards, 1996.

38. Doll et al., 1992.

39. Diamond, 2003c.

40. Savin-Williams, 2001b.

41. Savin-Williams & Ream, 2003b.

42. Hillier et al., 1998.

43. Russell & Joyner, 2001.

44. Rotheram-Borus et al., 1995, p. 83.

45. Diamond, 1998, 2000b, 2003b.

46. L. M. Diamond, personal communication, June 22, 2003.

47. Uribe & Harbeck, 1991, p. 12.

48. Hooker, 1957, p. 18.

49. Garofalo et al., 1998, 1999.

50. D'Augelli, Hershberger, & Pilkington, 2001; Remafedi et al., 1998; Rosario et al., 1996.

4. MODELS OR TRAJECTORIES?

1. Coleman, 1981–1982, pp. 32, 40; Cass, 1979, p. 219; Troiden, 1984, p. 105; Eliason, 1996b, p. 14, respectively.

2. Eliason, 1996b, Cox & Gallois, 1996, Fassinger & Miller, 1996, Horowitz & Newcomb, 2001, Morris, 1997, respectively.

3. Erikson, 1968, p. 50.

4. Ibid., p. 92.

5. Ibid., p. 174.

6. Ibid., pp. 96, 92.

7. Cass, 1979, 1983–1984, 1990.

8. McConnell, 1994.

9. Eliason, 1996a; Garnets & Kimmel, 1993; Horowitz & Newcomb, 2001; McConnell, 1994; Savin-Williams, 1998a, 2001a; Schneider, 2001, Suppe, 1984.

10. Coleman, 1981–1982.

11. Troiden, 1984.

12. Cass, 1979, pp. 220, 235.

13. Eliason, 1996a, p. 53.

14. Brown, 1995, p. 19.

15. Kitzinger & Wilkinson, 1995, p. 102.

16. Collins, 2000; Eliason, 1996a; Diamond & Savin-Williams, 2000; Tolman & Diamond, 2001.

17. Eliason, 1996b, Diamond, 1998, 2000b, 2003b; Gonsiorek, 1995.

18. Rust, 1992, 1993.

19. Faderman, 1984, p. 86.

20. Kitzinger & Wilkinson, 1995.

21. Gonsiorek, 1995.

22. Dubé, 2000.

23. Espin, 1987.

24. Manalansan, 1996, p. 410; Greene, 1994.

25. Chan, 1989, 1995; Icard, 1985–1986; Johnson, 1982.

26. Johnson, 1982.

27. Denizat-Lewis, 2003, p. 31.

28. Dubé & Savin-Williams, 1999.

29. Wooden, Kawasaki, & Mayeda, 1983.

30. Sophie, 1985–1986.

31. Savin-Williams, 1998a.

32. Diamond, 1998, 2000b, 2003b; see also Golden, 1996.

33. Savin-Williams, 1998a.

34. Weinberg, 1984, p. 81.

35. Brown, 1995, p. 17; Eliason, 1996a.

36. Collins, 2000; Weinberg, 1984; Brown, 1995, p. 18; Rust, 1992, 1993.

37. Frankel, 2003.

38. Weinberg, 1984, p. 78.

39. Steinberg, 1995.

40. Savin-Williams, 1998a, 2001b; Savin-Williams & Diamond, 1999.

41. Savin-Williams, 1990; Hillier et al., 1998; Diamond & Lucas, 2002.

42. Savin-Williams, 2001c; Savin-Williams & Ream, 2003b.

43. Shaffer et al., 1995.

44. Cohen, 1999, 2002, in press; Ellis, 1996a, 1996b; Hershberger, 1998.

45. Mustanski, Chivers, & Bailey, 2002; Rahman & Wilson, 2003.

46. Bogaert, Friesen, & Klentrou, 2002, p. 78; Savin-Williams & Ream, in preparation–b.

47. Hillier et al, 1998; Russell, 2002; Szalacha, 2001.

48. D'Augelli & Grossman, 2001; D'Augelli, Hershberger, & Pilkington, 2001.

49. Examples are available in Diamond & Dubé, 2002; Dubé, Savin-Williams, & Diamond, 2001.

50. Dubé & Savin-Williams, 1999; Manalansan, 1996.

51. Szalacha, 2001.

52. Russell, 2002.

53. Several of these examples are provided in Diamond, 1998.

5. FEELING DIFFERENT

1. Ellis, 1996a, 1996b.

2. Hanson & Hartmann, 1996.

3. Bailey, 1996; Bailey & Zucker, 1995.

4. Hanson & Hartmann, 1996.

5. Troiden, 1979.

6. Bell, Weinberg, & Hammersmith, 1981; also Troiden, 1979.

7. Troiden, 1979, 1989.

8. Schneider, 2001.

9. Saghir & Robbins, 1973.

10. D'Augelli & Grossman, 2001.

11. Ellis, 1901; Freud, 1905; Hirschfeld, 2000; Kennedy, 1988; Krafft-Ebing, 1922.

12. Chauncey, 1994.

13. Williams, 1996, pp. 421–422.

14. Bailey & Zucker, 1995; Meyer-Bahlburg, 1984.
15. Peplau et al., 1999, p. 71.
16. Sandfort, 2003; Terman & Miles, 1936.
17. S. Bem, 1974; Spence & Helmreich, 1978.
18. Green, 1987.
19. Bailey, 1996; Bailey & Zucker, 1995.
20. Grellert, Newcomb, & Bentler, 1982.
21. Diamond, 1998, 2003b.
22. Peplau et al., 1999, p. 83.
23. Bell, Weinberg, & Hammersmith, 1981.
24. Peplau et al., 1999.
25. Bailey & Zucker, 1995.
26. Phillips & Over, 1992, 1995.
27. Bailey & Zucker, 1995.
28. Bailey, Bechtold, & Berenbaum, 2002.
29. Savin-Williams, 1998a.
30. Bell, Weinberg, & Hammersmith, 1981.
31. Bailey & Zucker, 1995.
32. Hockenberry & Billingham, 1987, p. 485.
33. Grellert, Newcomb, & Bentler, 1982.
34. Ibid.
35. Bailey & Zucker, 1995.
36. Singh et al., 1999.
37. Phillips & Over, 1992, 1995.
38. Cohen, 2002.
39. D. Bem, 1996, 2001.
40. Peplau et al., 1999.
41. Bailey & Zucker, 1995.
42. Bailey, Miller, & Willerman, 1993.
43. Savin-Williams, 1998a, p. 35.
44. Troiden, 1989.

6. SAME-SEX ATTRACTIONS

1. Levine, 2002, pp. xix, 225.
2. Savin-Williams & Diamond, 2004.
3. Ibid.
4. Kinsey, Pomeroy, & Martin 1948; Kinsey et al., 1953.
5. Savin-Williams, in preparation.

6. D'Augelli & Grossman, 2001; see also Rosario et al., 1996.
7. Pattatucci & Hamer, 1995.
8. Ibid.
9. Herdt & McClintock, 2000; McClintock & Herdt, 1996.
10. Savin-Williams, in preparation.
11. Ibid.
12. D'Augelli, 1991a.
13. Dennis, 2002.
14. Savin-Williams, in preparation.
15. Baumeister, 2000.
16. Baumeister, Catanese, & Vosh, 2001; Knoth, Boyd, & Singer, 1988; Savin-Williams & Diamond, 2000, 2004; Rosario et al., 1996.
17. Rosario et al., 1996.
18. Savin-Williams, 1990.
19. Savin-Williams, in preparation.
20. Savin-Williams & Diamond, 2000.
21. Diamond, 2003c.
22. Knoth, Boyd, & Singer, 1988.
23. Savin-Williams, interview, February 1996.
24. Herdt & Boxer, 1993.
25. Hillier et al., 1998; Rosario et al., 1996; Storms, 1981.
26. Peplau et al., 1999.
27. Savin-Williams, in preparation.
28. Peplau et al., 1999, p. 90.
29. Savin-Williams, in preparation.
30. Golden, 1996; Weinberg, Williams, & Pryor, 1994.
31. Regan & Berscheid, 1995.
32. Savin-Williams, 1998a; Savin-Williams & Diamond, 2000.

7. FIRST SEX

1. Kinsey, Pomeroy, & Martin, 1948; Kinsey et al., 1953.
2. Kinsey, Pomeroy, & Martin, 1948, p. 168.
3. Kinsey et al., 1953.
4. Larsson & Svedin, 2002; Friedrich et al., 1991.
5. Larsson & Svedin, 2002.
6. Friedrich et al., 1991.
7. Okami, Olmstead, & Abramson, 1997; Larsson & Svedin, 2002.

8. Bauserman & Davis, 1996; Rind, 2001; Sandfort, 1992; Savin-Williams, 1998a.

9. Okami, Olmstead, & Abramson, 1997.

10. Ibid.

11. Roesler & Deisher, 1972, p. 1019.

12. Savin-Williams, 1998a, p. 90.

13. Ibid.

14. Ibid., pp. 90–91.

15. Savin-Williams, in preparation.

16. Kryzan, 1997.

17. Remafedi et al., 1992.

18. Hillier et al., 1998.

19. D'Augelli & Hershberger, 1993; D'Augelli, 1991a.

20. Garofalo et al., 1998.

21. Herek, 2004.

22. D'Augelli, 1991a; D'Augelli & Hershberger, 1993; DuRant, Krowchuk, & Sinal, 1998; Edwards, 1996; Faulkner & Cranston, 1998; Garofalo et al., 1998; Garofalo et al., 1999; Goode & Haber, 1977; Hillier et al., 1998; Kryzan, 1997, 2000; Remafedi, 1987b; Remafedi et al., 1992; Roesler & Deisher, 1972; Rosario et al., 1996; Rotheram-Borus, Hunter, & Rosario, 1994; Saewyc et al., 1998; Sears, 1991.

23. Herdt & Boxer, 1993.

24. Savin-Williams, in preparation.

25. Ibid.

26. D'Augelli, 1998.

27. D'Augelli & Hershberger, 1993; Herdt & Boxer, 1991; Roesler & Deisher, 1972; Rosario et al., 1996.

28. Baumeister, 2000; Diamond, in press; Weinberg, Williams, & Pryor, 1994.

29. Savin-Williams, in preparation.

30. Savin-Williams, 1998a; Savin-Williams & Diamond, 2004.

31. Roesler & Deisher, 1972.

32. Rotheram-Borus, Hunter, & Rosario, 1994.

33. Rosario et al., 1999.

34. D'Augelli, 1991a.

35. DuRant, Krowchuk, & Sinal, 1998.

36. Savin-Williams & Diamond, 2004.

37. Rosario et al., 1999.

38. Remafedi et al., 1992.
39. Mustanski, 2003; Sanders & Reinisch, 1999; Savin-Williams & Diamond, 2004.
40. Rotheram-Borus, Hunter, & Rosario, 1994.
41. Ibid.
42. Rosario et al., 1999.
43. Kryzan, 1997.
44. Goode & Haber, 1977.
45. Savin-Williams, 1998a, in preparation.
46. Savin-Williams, 1998a, p. 74.
47. Herdt & Boxer, 1993, p. 188.
48. Sears, 1991.
49. Ehrhardt, 1996.
50. Kryzan, 1997.
51. Savin-Williams & Diamond, 2004.
52. Rosario et al., 1999.
53. Kryzan, 2000.
54. Herdt & Boxer, 1993, p. 188.
55. Herdt & Boxer, 1993.
56. Kryzan, 1997, 2000.
57. Diamond, 1998; Savin-Williams & Diamond, 2000.
58. Savin-Williams & Diamond, 2004.
59. Rosario et al., 1996.
60. Savin-Williams & Diamond, 2004.

8. IDENTITY

1. Savin-Williams, in preparation.
2. Cass, 1979, 1983–1984, 1996.
3. Troiden, 1979.
4. Ibid.
5. Savin-Williams, 1998a, p. 54.
6. Diamond, 2003b.
7. Savin-Williams, in preparation.
8. Rosario et al., 1996.
9. Herdt & Boxer, 1993.
10. Telljohann & Price, 1993.
11. Savin-Williams, in preparation.

12. Herdt & Boxer, 1993, p. 210.
13. Roesler & Deisher, 1972; Remafedi, 1987a, 1987b.
14. Dubé, 2000.
15. Remafedi, 1987a.
16. Hillier et al., 1998.
17. Kryzan, 2000.
18. Ibid.
19. Diamond, 1998; Herdt & Boxer, 1993; Rosario et al., 1996; Savin-Williams & Diamond, 2000.
20. Diamond, 2003c; Dubé, 2000; Peplau et al., 1999; Schneider, 2001; Udry & Billy, 1987; Udry, Talbert, & Morris, 1986.
21. Dubé & Savin-Williams, 1999; Edwards, 1996.
22. D'Augelli, 1998; D'Augelli & Grossman, 2001; D'Augelli & Hershberger, 1993; Sears, 1991.
23. Savin-Williams, 2001a.
24. For reviews of this literature, see Savin-Williams, 1994, 2001c; Savin-Williams & Ream, 2003b.
25. Sears, 1991.
26. D'Augelli & Grossman, 2001; Hillier et al., 1998; Kryzan, 1997, 2000.
27. D'Augelli & Grossman, 2001; Savin-Williams, 2001b; Savin-Williams & Ream, 2003a.
28. Weeks, 1995, p. 44.
29. Savin-Williams & Diamond, 2000.
30. Rodríguez Rust, 2001.
31. Savin-Williams, in preparation; Rodríguez Rust, 2001.
32. Hillier et al., 1998.
33. Weinberg, Williams, & Pryor, 1994; Collins, 2000.
34. Herdt & Boxer, 1993, pp. 199, 201; Herdt, 2001, p. 277.
35. Rosario et al., 1996.
36. Rodríguez Rust, 2000, 2002, p. 185.
37. Rodríguez Rust, 2001, p. 66.
38. Hillier et al., 1998, p. 27.
39. Rust, 1993, Rodríguez Rust, 2001, p. 42; 2002.
40. Savin-Williams, in preparation.
41. Buzwell & Rosenthal, 1996.
42. Worthington et al., 2002, p. 496.
43. Two recent attempts to do this are Mohr, 2002 and Worthington et al., 2002.

44. Diamond, 2003c; Rodríguez Rust, 2002.
45. Eliason, 1995.
46. Frankel, 2003.
47. Ibid.

9. RESILIENCE AND DIVERSITY

1. Meyer, 2003, p. 685.
2. Savin-Williams & Ream, 2003b.
3. Orenstein, 2001.
4. Hillier et al., 1998, p. 31.
5. Ryan, 2000.
6. Savin-Williams, 2001b.
7. Porter, 2001; Smith, 2001.
8. Savin-Williams, 1990, 1998a, 2001c.
9. Clark et al., 1996; Luthar, Cicchetti, & Becker, 2000; Rutter, 1987.
10. Boxer & Cohler, 1989, p. 319.
11. D'Augelli, 1991b, p. 225.
12. McDaniel, Purcell, & D'Augelli, 2001; Remafedi, 1999a; Savin-Williams, 2001a.
13. Russell & Joyner, 2001; Savin-Williams, 2001c.
14. Hillier et al., 1998, p. 36.
15. Savin-Williams, 1998a, in preparation.
16. Russell, Seif, & Truong, 2001.
17. Edwards, 1996, p. 245.
18. Horowitz, Weis, & Laflin, 2001.
19. Peterson, Folkman, & Bakeman, 1996.
20. Healy, 2002.
21. Peterson & Bedogne, 2003.
22. Alexander, 1999, pp. 287, 289.
23. Ibid.
24. Sears, 1991; Herdt & Boxer, 1993; Rodríguez Rust, 2001, 2002.
25. Adam, 2000.
26. Hewitt, 1998.
27. Schneider, 2001.
28. Ibid., p. 79.
29. Tolman & Diamond, 2001, p. 52.
30. Fine, 1988; Tolman, 2002.

31. Tolman & Diamond, 2001, p. 62.
32. Diamond, 1998, 2000b, 2003b.
33. Diamond & Savin-Williams, 2000.
34. Rodríguez Rust, 2000.
35. Ibid., p. 215.
36. Russell, Bohan, & Lilly, 2000; Savin-Williams, 1990.
37. LaBarbera, 1994.
38. Savin-Williams, 1990, pp. 182, 185.

10. REFUSING AND RESISTING SEXUAL IDENTITY LABELS

1. Duberman, 2004, p. 22.
2. Schulman, 2004.
3. Hattersley, 2004, p. 33.
4. Ibid., p. 34.
5. Holleran, 2004, p. 12.
6. Ibid.
7. D'Emilio, 1983.
8. Ibid.; Savin-Williams & Diamond, 1997, pp. 218–219.
9. Kramer, 1997, p. 70.
10. Ibid., pp. 67, 70.
11. Signorile, 1999, pp. 73, 75.
12. Bronski, 1998; Weeks, 1995.
13. D'Emilio, 1999, all quotes p. 48.
14. Quoted in Champagne, 2003.
15. Reuters News Service, 2003.
16. Quoted in A. Cohen, 2003.
17. Cohen, 2003, p. 50.
18. D'Erasmo, 2004.
19. Goodridge, 2003.
20. Epstein, 2002a.
21. Epstein, 2002b.
22. Shaikin, 2000.
23. Ibid.
24. Stukin, 2002.
25. Lynch, 2002.
26. Shaikin, 2000.
27. Irvine, 2002.

28. Gdula, 2000.
29. Dukowitz, 2003.
30. Whoriskey, 2003.
31. Flocker, 2003.
32. Lipsky, 1998.
33. Dixit, 2001.
34. Ibid.
35. Quoted in Minzesheimer, 2000, p. 2D.
36. Bawer, 1993.
37. Lippa, 2000.
38. Fergusson, Horwood, & Beautrais, 1999; Meyer, 2003.
39. Savin-Williams, 1994.
40. Savin-Williams, unpublished interview.
41. Savin-Williams, in preparation.
42. Savin-Williams, 1998a, p. 135.
43. Savin-Williams, in preparation.
44. Steinberg, 1995.
45. Savin-Williams & Diamond, 2004.
46. Orenstein, 2001.
47. Lock & Steiner, 1999a.
48. Chauncey, 1994.
49. Herdt & Boxer, 1993, p. 202.
50. Muehlenhard, 2000.
51. Savin-Williams, in preparation.
52. Green, 1998, p. 91.
53. D'Erasmo, 2001, p. 106.
54. Kanner, 2003, p. 34.
55. Bahr, 2001, pp. 74, 70, 72.
56. Bauder, 2002, p. 42.
57. Champagne, 2001.
58. Hillier et al., 1998, p. 26; D'Erasmo, 2001, pp. 104, 106.
59. D'Erasmo, 2001.
60. Rodríguez Rust, 2001, 2002; Rothblum, 2000.
61. Laan, Sonderman, & Janssen, 1996.
62. Chivers et al., 2004.
63. Pattatucci & Hamer, 1995; Rodríguez Rust, 2000, 2001; Rothblum, 2000; Schneider, 2001; Weinberg, Williams, & Pryor, 1994.
64. Savin-Williams, in preparation.

65. Diamond, 2003b, p. 360.
66. Tolman & Diamond, 2001, p. 61.
67. Diamond, 2003b, pp. 361–362.
68. Tolman & Diamond, 2001, p. 61.
69. Cardoso & Werner, 2004, p. 204.
70. Scalia, 2003, p. E2.
71. Tofiño, 2003, p. 18.
72. Denizet-Lewis, 2003, p. 30.
73. Ibid., p. 31.
74. Bergman, 2004, p. 17.
75. McConaghy, 1999, p. 296.
76. Diamond, 2003a, p. 86.
77. Duralde, 2002b, p. 53.
78. Duralde, 2002a, p. 44.
79. Gottman et al., 2003a, 2003b.
80. Gottman et al., 2003b, p. 88.
81. DiPlacido, 1998, pp. 139, 148; see also Meyer, 2003; Sandfort, 1997.
82. Levey, 2002.
83. From, respectively, *The Advocate,* June 19, 2001, p. 15, and April 5, 1994, p. 35; *Washington Post,* October 24, 1988, p. A1; *Cleveland Plain Dealer,* April 6, 1997, p. 1A; *Texas Triangle,* July 21, 1993; *Raleigh News and Observer,* June 30, 2000, p. 1; and *Out,* July 2001, p. 38.
84. Dineen, 1996.
85. Bronski, 1998, pp. 48–49.
86. Tolman & Diamond, 2001, p. 61.
87. Weeks, 1995, p. 44.
88. Alexander, 1999, p. 289.
89. James, 1999.

References

Adam, B. D. (2000). Love and sex in constructing identity among men who have sex with men. *International Journal of Sexuality and Gender Studies, 5,* 325–339.

Alexander, J. (1999). Introduction to the special issue: Queer values, beyond identity. *Journal of Gay, Lesbian, and Bisexual Identity, 4,* 287–292.

Associated Press (2003a, July 2). Wal-Mart adds gays to workplace policy. Pulled from Earthlink's news.

Associated Press (2003b, June 26). Supreme Court strikes down Texas law banning sodomy. *New York Times.* www.nytimes.com/2003/06/p . . . / 26WIRE-SODO.html.

Associated Press (2003c, September 30). Episcopal head defends choice of gay bishop. *New York Times.* www.nytimes.com/2003/09/03/national/ 30BISH.html.

Bahr, D. (2001, January 16). This boy's life. *The Advocate,* pp. 68–75.

Bailey, J. M. (1996). Gender identity. In R. C. Savin-Williams & K. M. Cohen (Eds.), *The lives of lesbians, gays, and bisexuals: Children to adults* (pp. 71–93). Fort Worth, TX: Harcourt Brace College Publishing.

Bailey, J. M., Bechtold, K. T., & Berenbaum, S. A. (2002). Who are tomboys and why should we study them? *Archives of Sexual Behavior, 31,* 333–341.

Bailey, J. M., Miller, J. S., & Willerman, L. (1993). Maternally related childhood gender nonconformity in homosexuals and heterosexuals. *Archives of Sexual Behavior, 22,* 461–469.

Bailey, J. M., & Zucker, K. J. (1995). Childhood sex-typed behavior and sexual orientation: A conceptual analysis and quantitative review. *Developmental Psychology, 31*, 43–55.

Battle, C. (1998, February). *Sexual identity development among ethnic/sexual minority males.* Paper presented at the Seventh Biennial Meeting of the Society for Research on Adolescence, San Diego.

Bauder, D. (2002, March 27). Rosie O'Donnell says being gay was "never a big deal for me." *In Newsweekly, 11/31*, p. 42.

Baumeister, R. F. (2000). Gender differences in erotic plasticity: The female sex drive as socially flexible and responsive. *Psychological Bulletin, 126*, 247–374.

Baumeister, R. F., Catanese, K. R., & Vohs, K. D. (2001). Is there a gender difference in strength of sex drive? Theoretical views, conceptual distinctions, and a review of relevant evidence. *Personality and Social Psychology Review, 5*, 242–273.

Bauserman, R., & Davis C. (1996). Perceptions of early sexual experiences and adult sexual adjustment. *Journal of Psychology and Human Sexuality, 8*, 37–59.

Bawer, B. (1993). *A place at the table: The gay individual in American society.* New York: Poseidon Press.

Bell, A. P., Weinberg, M. S., & Hammersmith, S. K. (1981). *Sexual preference: Its development in men and women.* Bloomington: Indiana University Press.

Bem, D. J. (1996). Exotic becomes erotic: A developmental theory of sexual orientation. *Psychological Review, 103*, 320–335.

Bem, D. J. (2001). Exotic becomes erotic: Integrating biological and experiential antecedents of sexual orientation. In A. R. D'Augelli & C. J. Patterson (Eds.), *Lesbian, gay, and bisexual identities and youth: Psychological perspectives* (pp. 52–68). New York: Oxford University Press.

Bem, S. L. (1974). The measurement of psychological androgyny. *Journal of Consulting and Clinical Psychology, 42*, 165–172.

Bergman, D. (2004, January–February). Please pass the pepper. *The Gay and Lesbian Review, 11*, pp. 17–19.

Bogaert, A. F., & Fisher, W. A. (1995). Predictors of university men's number of sexual partners. *Journal of Sex Research, 32*, 119–131.

Bogaert, A. F., Friesen, C., & Klentrou, P. (2002). Age of puberty and sexual orientation in a national probability sample. *Archives of Sexual Behavior, 31*, 73–81.

Boxer, A. M., & Cohler, B. J. (1989). The life course of gay and lesbian youth:

An immodest proposal for the study of lives. *Journal of Homosexuality, 17,* 315–355.

Brady, S., & Busse, W. J. (1994). The Gay Identity Questionnaire: A brief measure of homosexual identity formation. *Journal of Homosexuality, 26,* 1–22.

Bronski, M. (1998). *The pleasure principle: Sex, backlash, and the struggle for gay freedom.* New York: St. Martin's Press.

Brown, J. D. (2002). Mass media influences on sexuality. *Journal of Sex Research, 39,* 42–45.

Brown, L. S. (1995). Lesbian identities: Concepts and issues. In A. R. D'Augelli & C. J. Patterson (Eds.), *Lesbian, gay, and bisexual identities over the lifespan: Psychological perspectives* (pp. 3–23). New York: Oxford University Press.

Bullough, V., & Bullough, B. (1980). Homosexuality in nineteenth century English public schools. In J. Harry & M. S. Das (Eds.), *Homosexuality in international perspective* (pp. 123–131). New Delhi: Vikas.

Buzwell, S., & Rosenthal, D. (1996). Constructing a sexual self: Adolescents' sexual self-perceptions and sexual risk-taking. *Journal of Research on Adolescence, 6,* 489–513.

Carballo-Diéguez, A. (1997). Sexual research with Latino men who have sex with men. In J. Bancroft (Ed.), *Researching sexual behavior: Methodological issues* (pp. 134–144). Bloomington: Indiana University Press.

Cardoso, F. L., & Werner, D. (2004). Homosexuality. In C. R. Ember & M. Ember (Eds.), *Encyclopedia of sex and gender: Men and women in the world's cultures* (Vol. 1) (pp. 204–215). New York: Kluwer Academic/ Plenum.

Carpenter, L. M. (2001). The ambiguity of "having sex": The subjective experience of virginity loss in the United States. *Journal of Sex Research, 38,* 127–139.

Carrier, J. (1995). *De los ostros: Intimacy and homosexuality among Mexican men.* New York: Columbia University Press.

Cass, V. (1979). Homosexual identity formation: A theoretical model. *Journal of Homosexuality, 4,* 219–235.

Cass, V. (1983/1984). Homosexual identity: A concept in need of a definition. *Journal of Homosexuality, 9,* 105–126.

Cass, V. C. (1990). The implications of homosexual identity formation for the Kinsey Model and Scale of Sexual Preference. In D. P. McWhirter, S. A. Sanders, & J. M. Reinisch (Eds.), *Homosexuality/heterosexuality: Concepts of sexual orientation* (pp. 239–266). New York: Oxford University Press.

Cass, V. (1996). Sexual orientation identity formation: A Western phenomenon. In R. P. Cabaj & T. S. Stein, eds., *Textbook of homosexuality and mental health* (pp. 227–251). Washington, DC: American Psychiatric Press.

Catlin, R. (2004, January 20). "The Daily Show" gears up for election. From the *Hartford Courier* as reported in *Fayetteville Observer* (NC), p. 3E.

Champagne, C. (2001, August). On the road. *Out*, p. 30.

Champagne, C. (2003, September 4). "Gaywatch: The dish from James of "Boy Meets Boy." Retrieved from www.planetout.com/entertainment/news/splash.

Chan, C. S. (1989). Issues of identity development among Asian-American lesbians and gay men. *Journal of Counseling and Development, 68,* 16–20.

Chan, C. S. (1995). Issues of sexual identity in an ethnic minority: The case of Chinese American lesbians, gay men, and bisexual people. In A. R. D'Augelli & C. J. Patterson (Eds.), *Lesbian, gay, and bisexual identities over the lifespan: Psychological perspectives* (pp. 87–101). New York: Oxford University Press.

Chauncey, G. (1994). *Gay New York: Gender, urban culture, and the making of the gay male world, 1890–1940.* New York: Basic Books.

Chivers, M. L., Rieger, G., Latty, E., & Bailey, J. M. (2004). A sex difference in the specificity of sexual arousal. *Psychological Science, 15,* 736–744.

Chung, Y. B., & Katayama, M. (1996). Assessment of sexual orientation in lesbian/gay/bisexual studies. *Journal of Homosexuality, 30,* 49–62.

Clark, L., Marsh, G. W., Davis, M., Igoe, J., & Stember, M. (1996). Adolescent health promotion in a low-income, urban environment. *Family Community Health, 19,* 1–13.

Cohen, A. (2003, November–December). Eyes on the guys: Gay men's turn on TV. *Gay and Lesbian Review, 10,* 50.

Cohen, K. M. (1999). *The biology of male sexual orientation: Relationship among homoeroticism, childhood sex-atypical behavior, spatial ability, handedness, and pubertal timing.* Unpublished doctoral dissertation, University of Detroit Mercy, Detroit.

Cohen, K. M. (2002). Relationships among childhood sex-atypical behavior, spatial ability, handedness, and sexual orientation in men. *Archives of Sexual Behavior, 31,* 129–143.

Cohen, K. M. (in press). Etiology of homoeroticism. In E. Perrin (Ed.), *Current problems in pediatric and adolescent health care.*

Cohen, K. M., & Savin-Williams, R. C. (1996). Developmental perspectives on coming out to self and others. In R. C. Savin-Williams & K. M. Cohen (Eds.), *The lives of lesbians, gays, and bisexuals: Children to adults* (pp. 113–151). Forth Worth, TX: Harcourt Brace College Publishing.

Cohler, B. J., & Galatzer-Levy, R. M. (2000). *The course of gay and lesbian lives: Social and psychoanalytic perspectives.* Chicago: University of Chicago Press.

Coleman, E. (1981–1982). Developmental stages of the coming out process. *Journal of Homosexuality, 7,* 31–43.

Coleman, E. (1990). Toward a synthetic understanding of sexual orientation. In D. P. McWhirter, S. A. Sanders, & J. M. Reinisch (Eds.), *Homosexuality/ heterosexuality: Concepts of sexual orientation* (pp. 267–276). New York: Oxford University Press.

Collard, J. (2000, January). Pet Shop Boys. *Out,* pp. 40–43, 89.

Collins, J. F. (2000). Biracial-bisexual individuals: Identity coming of age. *International Journal of Sexuality and Gender Studies, 5,* 221–253.

Copas, A. J., Wellings, K., Erens, B., Mercer, C. H., McManus, S., Fenton, K. A., Korovessis, C., Macdowall, W., Nanchahal, K., & Johnson, A. M. (2002). The accuracy of reported sensitive sexual behaviour in Britain: Exploring the extent of change, 1990–2000. *Sexual Transmission and Infection, 78,* 26–30.

Cox, S., & Gallois, C. (1996). Gay and lesbian identity development: A social identity perspective. *Journal of Homosexuality, 30,* 1–30.

D'Augelli, A. R. (1991a). Gay men in college: Identity processes and adaptations. *Journal of College Student Development, 32,* 140–146.

D'Augelli, A. R. (1991b). Teaching lesbian/gay development: From oppression to exceptionality. *Journal of Homosexuality, 22,* 213–227.

D'Augelli, A. R. (1998, February). Victimization history and mental health among lesbian, gay, and bisexual youths. Paper presented at the biennial meetings of the Society for Research on Adolescence, San Diego, CA.

D'Augelli, A. R., & Grossman, A. H. (2001, August). Sexual orientation victimization of lesbian, gay, and bisexual youths. Paper presented at the American Psychological Association, San Francisco.

D'Augelli, A. R., & Hershberger, S. L. (1993). Lesbian, gay, and bisexual youth in community settings: Personal challenges and mental health problems. *American Journal of Community Psychology, 21,* 421–448.

D'Augelli, A. R., Hershberger, S. L., & Pilkington, N. W. (2001). Suicidality patterns and sexual orientation-related factors among lesbian, gay, and bisexual youths. *Suicide and Life-Threatening Behavior, 31,* 250–264.

D'Emilio, J. (1983). *Sexual politics, sexual communities: The making of a homosexual minority in the United States, 1940–1970.* Chicago: University of Chicago Press.

D'Emilio, J. (1999, Winter). The gaying of America. *Harvard Gay and Lesbian Review, 6,* 48–49.

D'Emilio, J. (2002). *The world turned: Essays on gay history, politics, and culture.* Durham, NC: Duke University Press.

D'Emilio, J., & Freedman, E. B. (1988). *Intimate matters: A history of sexuality in America.* New York: Harper & Row.

Denizet-Lewis, B. (2003, August 3). Double lives on the down low. *New York Times Magazine* pp. 28–33, 48, 52–53.

Dennis, J. (2002, December 4). Retrieved from http://wise.fau.edu/jdennis/gaytv.

D'Erasmo, S. (2001, October 14). Polymorphous normal: Has sexual identity—gay, straight or bi—outlived its usefulness? *New York Times Magazine,* pp. 104–107.

D'Erasmo, S. (2004, January 11). Lesbians on TV: It's not easy being seen. *New York Times,* Arts & Leisure, p. 1.

Diamond, L. M. (1998). The development of sexual orientation among adolescent and young adult women. *Developmental Psychology, 34,* 1085–1095.

Diamond, L. M. (2000a). Passionate friendships among adolescent sexual-minority women. *Journal of Research on Adolescence, 10,* 191–209.

Diamond, L. M. (2000b). Sexual identity, attractions, and behavior among young sexual-minority women over a two-year period. *Developmental Psychology, 36,* 241–250.

Diamond, L. M. (2003a). Love matters: Romantic relationships among sexual-minority adolescents. In P. Florsheim (Ed.), *Adolescent romantic relations and sexual behavior: Theory, research, and practical implications* (pp. 85–107). Mahwah, NJ: Lawrence Erlbaum.

Diamond, L. M. (2003b). Was it a phase? Young women's relinquishment of lesbian/bisexual identities over a five-year period. *Journal of Personality and Social Psychology, 84,* 352–364.

Diamond, L. M. (2003c). What does sexual orientation orient? A biobehavioral model distinguishing romantic love and sexual desire. *Psychological Review, 110,* 173–192.

Diamond, L. M. (in press). What we got wrong about sexual identity development: Unexpected findings from a longitudinal study of young women. In

A. Omoto & H. Kurtzman (Eds.), *Recent research on sexual orientation.* Washington, DC: American Psychological Association.

Diamond, L. M., & Dubé, E. M. (2002). Friendship and attachment among heterosexual and sexual-minority youths: Does the gender of your friend matter? *Journal of Youth and Adolescence, 31,* 155–166.

Diamond, L. M., & Lucas, S. (2002, April). Close relationships and well-being among sexual-minority and heterosexual youths. Paper presented at the Society for Research on Adolescence, New Orleans, LA.

Diamond, L. M., & Savin-Williams, R. C. (2000). Explaining diversity in the development of same-sex sexuality among young women. *Journal of Social Issues, 56,* 297–313.

Diamond, M. (1993). Homosexuality and bisexuality in different populations. *Archives of Sexual Behavior, 22,* 291–310.

Dineen, T. (1996). *Manufacturing victims: What the psychology industry is doing to people.* Montreal: Robert Davies.

DiPlacido, J. (1998). Minority stress among lesbians, gay men, and bisexuals: A consequence of heterosexism, homophobia, and stigmatization. In G. M. Herek (Ed.), *Psychological perspectives on lesbian and gay issues: Vol. 4. Stigma and sexual orientation: Understanding prejudice against lesbians, gay men, and bisexuals* (pp. 138–159). Thousand Oaks, CA: Sage.

Dixit, J. (2001, October 11). To be gay at Yale. *Rolling Stone.* Retrieved from www.rollingstone.com/features/college/article.asp?id=7.

Dobinson, C. (1999). Confessions of an identity junkie. *Journal of Gay, Lesbian, and Bisexual Identity, 4,* 265–269.

Doll, L. S., Petersen, L. R., White, C. R., Johnson, E. S., Ward, J. W., & the Blood Donor Study Group (1992). Homosexually and nonhomosexually identified men who have sex with men: A behavioral comparison. *Journal of Sex Research, 29,* 1–14.

Dowd, M. (2003, August 3). Butch, butch Bush! *New York Times,* p. 11.

Dubé, E. M. (2000). The role of sexual behavior in the identification process of gay and bisexual males. *Journal of Sex Research, 37,* 123–132.

Dubé, E. M., & Savin-Williams, R. C. (1999). Sexual identity development among ethnic sexual-minority male youths. *Developmental Psychology, 35,* 1389–1399.

Dubé, E. M., Savin-Williams, R. C., & Diamond, L. M. (2001). Intimacy development, gender, and ethnicity among sexual-minority youths. In A. R. D'Augelli & C. J. Patterson (Eds.), *Lesbian, gay, and bisexual identities and youths: Psychological perspectives* (pp. 129–152). New York: Oxford University Press.

Duberman, M. (2004, January–February). The unmaking of a movement. *Gay and Lesbian Review, 11,* pp. 22–23.

Dukowitz, G. (2003, February 4). Virtually gay. *The Advocate,* p. 21.

Duralde, A. (2002a, October 29). A man's man. *The Advocate,* pp. 44–48.

Duralde, A. (2002b, October 29). Belle toujours. *The Advocate,* pp. 53–54.

DuRant, R. H., Krowchuk, D. P., & Sinal, S. H. (1998). Victimization, use of violence, and drug use at school among male adolescents who engage in same-sex sexual behavior. *Journal of Pediatrics, 132,* 113–118.

Edwards, W. J. (1996). Operating within the mainstream: Coping and adjustment among a sample of homosexual youths. *Deviant Behavior: An Interdisciplinary Journal, 17,* 229–251.

Ehrhardt, A. A. (1996). Our view of adolescent sexuality: A focus on risk behavior without the developmental context. *American Journal of Public Health, 86,* 1523–1525.

Eliason, M. J. (1995). Accounts of sexual identity formation in heterosexual students. *Sex Roles, 32,* 821–834.

Eliason, M. J. (1996a). Identity formation for lesbian, bisexual and gay persons: Beyond a "minoritizing" view. *Journal of Homosexuality, 30,* 31–58.

Eliason, M. J. (1996b). An inclusive model of lesbian identity assumption. *Journal of Gay, Lesbian, and Bisexual Identity, 1,* 3–19.

Ellis, H. (1901). *Studies in the psychology of sex: Vol. 2. Sexual inversion.* Philadelphia: F. A. Davis.

Ellis, L. (1996a). Theories of homosexuality. In R. C. Savin-Williams & K. M. Cohen (Eds.), *The lives of lesbians, gays, and bisexuals: Children to adults* (pp. 11–34). Fort Worth, TX: Harcourt Brace College Publishing.

Ellis, L. (1996b). The role of perinatal factors in determining sexual orientation. In R. C. Savin-Williams & K. M. Cohen (Eds.), *The lives of lesbians, gays, and bisexuals: Children to adults* (pp. 35–70). Fort Worth, TX: Harcourt Brace College Publishing.

Epstein, J. (2002a, January). Sensitive souls. *Out,* pp. 38–44.

Epstein, J. (2002b, May). Boston Public sex. *Out,* pp. 30–32.

Epstein, J. (2004, February). Daytime's newest diva. *Out,* pp. 37–41.

Erikson, E. H. (1968). *Identity: Youth and crisis.* New York: Norton.

Espin, O. M. (1987). Issues of identity in the psychology of Latina lesbians. In Boston Lesbian Psychologies Collective (Ed.), *Lesbian psychologies: Explorations and challenges* (pp. 35–55). Urbana: University of Illinois Press.

Faderman, L. (1977, September). Emily Dickinson's letters to Sue Gilbert. *Massachusetts Review, 18,* 19–27.

Faderman, L. (1981). *Surpassing the love of men: Romantic friendship and love between women from the Renaissance to the present.* New York: William Morrow.

Faderman, L. (1984). The "new gay" lesbians. *Journal of Homosexuality, 10,* 85–95.

Fassinger, R. E., & Miller, B. A. (1996). Validation of an inclusive model of sexual minority formation on a sample of gay men. *Journal of Homosexuality, 32,* 53–78.

Faulkner, A. H., & Cranston, K. (1998). Correlates of same-sex sexual behavior in a random sample of Massachusetts high school students. *American Journal of Public Health, 88,* 262–266.

Fergusson, D. M., Horwood, L. J., & Beautrais, A. L. (1999). Is sexual orientation related to mental health problems and suicidality in young people? *Archives of General Psychiatry, 56,* 876–880.

Fetto, J. (2001, June). Don't ask, don't tell. *American Demographics, 23*(6), p. 27.

Fine, M. (1988). Sexuality, schooling, and adolescent females: The missing discourse of desire. *Harvard Educational Review, 58,* 29–53.

Finn, R. (2004, March 25). This Queer Eye takes design to the masses. *New York Times,* p. B2.

Flocker, M. (2003). *The metrosexual guide to style: A handbook for the modern man.* Cambridge, MA: Da Capo Press.

Foucault, M. (1978). *The history of sexuality.* Translated by Robert Hurley. New York: Pantheon.

Fox, R. C. (1995). Bisexual identities. In A. R. D'Augelli & C. J. Patterson (Eds.), *Lesbian, gay, and bisexual identities over the lifespan: Psychological perspectives* (pp. 48–86). New York: Oxford University Press.

Frankel, L. B. (2003). *Do heterosexual men have a sexual identity? An exploratory study.* Unpublished doctoral dissertation, Cornell University, Ithaca, NY.

Freud, S. (1905). *Three essays on the theory of sexuality.* London: Imago.

Friedman, M. S., Silvestre, A. J., Gold, M. A., Markovic, N., Savin-Williams, R. C., Huggins, J., & Sell, R. L. (2004). Adolescents define sexual orientation and suggest ways to measure it. *Journal of Adolescence, 27,* 303–317.

Friedrich, W. N., Grambsch, P., Broughton, D., Kuiper, J., & Beilke, R. L. (1991). Normative sexual behavior in children. *Pediatrics, 88,* 456–464.

Gagnon, J. H., & Simon, W. (1973). *Sexual conduct: The social sources of human sexuality.* Chicago: Aldine.

Gangestad, S. W., Bailey, J. M., & Martin, N. G. (2000). Taxometric analyses of sexual orientation and gender identity. *Journal of Personality and Social Psychology, 78,* 1109–1121.

Garnets, L. D., & Kimmel, D. C. (1993). Introduction: Lesbian and gay male dimensions in the psychological study of human diversity. In L. D. Garnets & D. C. Kimmel (Eds.), *Psychological perspectives on lesbian and gay male experiences* (pp. 1–51). New York: Columbia University Press.

Garofalo, R., Wolf, R. C., Kessel, S., Palfrey, J., & DuRant, R. H. (1998). The association between health risk behaviors and sexual orientation among a school-based sample of adolescents. *Pediatrics, 101,* 895–902.

Garofalo, R., Wolf, R. C., Wissow, L. S., Woods, E. R., & Goodman, E. (1999). Sexual orientation and risk of suicide attempts among a representative sample of youth. *Archives of Pediatric Adolescent Medicine, 153,* 487–493.

Gdula, S. (2000, November 21). Double the power. *The Advocate,* p. 80.

Gideonse, T. (2001, December). Teen target. *Out,* pp. 17–19.

Golden, C. (1996). What's in a name? Sexual self-identification among women. In R. C. Savin-Williams & K. M. Cohen (Eds.), *The lives of lesbians, gays, and bisexuals: Children to adults* (pp. 229–249). Fort Worth, TX: Harcourt Brace College Publishing.

Gonsiorek, J. C. (1995). Gay male identities: Concepts and issues. In A. R. D'Augelli & C. J. Patterson (Eds.), *Lesbian, gay, and bisexual identities over the lifespan: Psychological perspectives* (pp. 24–47). New York: Oxford University Press.

Gonsiorek, J. C., Sell, R. L., & Weinrich, J. D. (1995). Definition and measurement of sexual orientation. *Suicide and Life-Threatening Behavior, 25* (Supplement), 40–51.

Goode, E., & Haber, L. (1977). Sexual correlates of homosexual experience: An exploratory study of college women. *Journal of Sex Research, 13,* 12–21.

Goodridge, M. (2003, April 1). Pre-Stonewall preteen. *The Advocate,* p. 52.

Gottman, J. M., Levenson, R. W., Gross, J., Frederickson, B. L., McCoy, K., Rosenthal, L., Ruef, A., & Yoshimoto, D. (2003a). Observing gay, lesbian and heterosexual couples' relationships: Mathematical modeling of conflict interaction. *Journal of Homosexuality, 45,* 23–43.

Gottman, J. M., Levenson, R. W., Swanson, C., Swanson, K., Tyson, R., & Yoshimoto, D. (2003b). Observing gay, lesbian and heterosexual couples' relationships: Mathematical modeling of conflict interaction. *Journal of Homosexuality, 45,* 65–91.

Green, B. C. (1998). Thinking about students who do not identify as gay, lesbian, or bisexual, but . . . *Journal of American College Health, 47,* 89–91.

Green, R. (1987). *The "sissy boy syndrome" and the development of homosexuality.* New Haven, CT: Yale University Press.

Greene, B. (1994). Ethnic-minority lesbians and gay men: Mental health and treatment issues. *Journal of Consulting Clinical Psychology, 62,* 243–251.

Grellert, E. A., Newcomb, M. D., & Bentler, P. M. (1982). Childhood play activities of male and female homosexuals and heterosexuals. *Archives of Sexual Behavior, 11,* 451–478.

Griffin, P., Lee, C., Waugh, J., & Beyer, C. (2004). Describing roles that gay-straight alliances play in schools: From individual support to school change. *Journal of Gay and Lesbian Issues in Education, 1,* 7–22.

Gross, J. J. (2000, August). The queen is dead: Once a gay icon, Judy Garland has become an embarrassment. *Atlantic Monthly.*

Hale, E. (2003, May 3). The most famous athlete in the world (except in the USA). *USA Today,* pp. 1–2.

Hall, C., & Simmons, K. (2001, June 26). Talking about sexual orientation. *USA Today,* p. 8D.

Halpern, C. T., Udry, J. R., Campbell, B., & Suchindran, C. (1993). Testosterone and pubertal development as predictors of sexual activity: A panel analysis of adolescent males. *Psychosomatic Medicine, 55,* 436–447.

Halpert, S. C. (2002). Suicidal behavior among gay male youth. *Journal of Gay and Lesbian Psychotherapy, 6,* 53–79.

Hamilton College & Zogby International (2001, August 28). High school seniors liberal on gay issues. *USA Today,* p. 8D.

Hanson, G., & Hartmann, L. (1996). Latency development in prehomosexual boys. In R. P. Cabaj & T. S. Stein (Eds.), *Textbook of homosexuality and mental health* (pp. 253–266). Washington, DC: American Psychiatric Press.

Harris, D. (1997). *The rise and fall of gay culture.* New York: Ballantine Books.

Hattersley, M. (2004, January–February). Will success spoil gay culture? *Gay and Lesbian Review, 11,* pp. 33–34.

Healy, P. (2002, May 21). College recruiters look to gays but schools see problem in identifying students. *Boston Globe.*

Hedblom, J. H., & Hartman, J. J. (1980). Research on lesbianism: Selected effects of time, geographic location, and data collection technique. *Archives of Sexual Behavior, 9,* 217–234.

Herdt, G. (1987). *The Sambia: Ritual and gender in New Guinea.* New York: Holt, Rinehart & Winston.

Herdt, G. (Ed.) (1989). *Gay and lesbian youth.* New York: Harrington Park Press.

Herdt, G. (2001). Social change, sexual diversity, and tolerance for bisexuality in the United States. In A. R. D'Augelli & C. J. Patterson (Eds.), *Lesbian, gay, and bisexual identities and youth: Psychological perspectives* (pp. 267–283). New York: Oxford University Press.

Herdt, G., & Boxer, A. M. (1993). *Children of Horizons: How gay and lesbian teens are leading a new way out of the closet.* Boston: Beacon Press.

Herdt, G., & McClintock, M. (2000). The magical age of 10. *Archives of Sexual Behavior, 29,* 587–606.

Herdt, G., Russell, S., Sweat, J., & Marzullo, M. (in preparation). *Sexual inequality, youth empowerment, and the GSA: A community study in California.* San Francisco State University, San Francisco, CA.

Herek, G. M. (2004). Beyond "homophobia": Thinking about sexual prejudice and stigma in the twenty-first century. *Sexual Research and Social Policy: Journal of NSRC, 1*(2), 6–24.

Hershberger, S. L. (1998). Homosexuality. In H. Friedman (Ed.), *Encyclopedia of mental health* (Vol. 2) (pp. 403–419). San Diego: Academic Press.

Hewitt, C. (1998). Homosexual demography: Implications for the spread of AIDS. *Journal of Sex Research, 35,* 390–396.

Hillier, L., Dempsey, D., Harrison, L., Beale, L. Matthews, L. & Rosenthal, D. (1998). *Writing themselves in: A national report on the sexuality, health and well-being of same-sex attracted young people.* Monograph series 7, Australian Research Centre in Sex, Health and Society, National Centre in HIV Social Research, La Trobe University, Carlton, Australia.

Hirschfeld, M. (2000). *The homosexuality of men and women.* Translated by M. A. Lombardi-Nash. Amherst, NY: Prometheus Books.

Hockenberry, S. L., & Billingham, R. E. (1987). Sexual orientation and boyhood gender conformity: Development of the Boyhood Gender Conformity Scale (BGCS). *Archives of Sexual Behavior, 16,* 475–492.

Holleran, A. (2004, January–February). The day after. *Gay and Lesbian Review, 11,* pp. 12–16.

Holmes, S. E., & Cahill, S. (2004). School experiences of gay, lesbian, bisexual, and transgender youth. *Journal of Gay and Lesbian Issues in Education, 1,* 53–60.

Hooker, E. A. (1957). The adjustment of the male overt homosexual. *Journal of Projective Techniques, 21,* 17–31.

Horowitz, J. L., & Newcomb, M. D. (2001). A multidimensional approach to homosexual identity. *Journal of Homosexuality, 42,* 1–19.

Horowitz, S. M., Weis, D. L., & Laflin, M. T. (2001). Differences between sexual orientation behavior groups and social background, quality of life, and health behaviors. *Journal of Sex Research, 38,* 205–218.

Icard, L. (1985–1986). Black gay men and conflicting social identities: Sexual orientation versus racial identity. *Journal of Social Work and Human Sexuality, 4,* 83–93.

Irvine, M. (2002, December 16). Two Illinois girls voted high school's "cutest couple." *Ithaca Journal,* p. 9.

James, A. (1999, Fall). In search of ordinary Joes. *McGill News,* p. 52.

Johnson, J. M. (1982). Influence of assimilation on the psychosocial adjustment of Black homosexual men. *Dissertation Abstracts International, 42*(11), 4620-B.

Jones, G. P. (1978). Counseling gay adolescents. *Counselor Education and Supervision, 18,* 149–152.

Journal of Gay and Lesbian Issues in Education (2004). Gay-straight alliances. Special issue, *1*(3).

Journal of Gay and Lesbian Issues in Education (in press). Resiliency. Special issue.

Kanner, M. (2003, July–August). Can *Will & Grace* be "queered"? *Gay and Lesbian Review, 10,* 34–35.

Kauth, M. R. (2002). Much ado about homosexuality: Assumptions underlying current research on sexual orientation. *Journal of Psychology and Human Sexuality, 14,* 1–22.

Kennedy, H. (1988). *The life and works of Karl Heinrich Ulrichs: Pioneer of the modern gay movement.* Boston: Alyson.

Kinsey, A. C., Pomeroy, W. B., & Martin, C. E. (1948). *Sexual behavior in the human male.* Philadelphia: W. B. Saunders.

Kinsey, A. C., Pomeroy, W. B., Martin, C. E., & Gebhard, P. H. (1953). *Sexual behavior in the human female.* Philadelphia: W. B. Saunders.

Kitzinger, C. (1987). *The social construction of lesbianism.* London: Sage.

Kitzinger, C., & Wilkinson, S. (1995). Transitions from heterosexuality to lesbianism: The discursive production of lesbian identities. *Developmental Psychology, 31,* 95–104.

Klein, F., Sepekoff, B., & Wolf, T. J. (1985). Sexual orientation: A multi-variable dynamic process. *Journal of Homosexuality, 11,* 35–49.

Knoth, R., Boyd, K., & Singer, B. (1988). Empirical tests of sexual selection theory: Predictions of sex differences in onset, intensity, and time course of sexual arousal. *Journal of Sex Research, 24,* 73–89.

Krafft-Ebing, R. von (1925). *Psychopathia sexualis: A medico-forensic study.* Translated by F. J. Rebman. Brooklyn, NY: Physicians and Surgeons.

Kramer, L. (1997, May 27). Sex and sensibility. *The Advocate,* pp. 59, 64–65, 67–70.

Krauss, C. (2003, August 31). Now free to marry, Canada's gays say, "Do I?" *New York Times,* pp. 1, 14.

Kryzan, C. (1997). OutProud/Oasis Internet Survey of Queer and Questioning Youth. Sponsored by OutProud, The National Coalition for Gay, Lesbian, Bisexual and Transgender Youth and *Oasis Magazine.* Contact survey@outproud.org.

Kryzan, C. (2000). OutProud/Oasis Internet Survey of Queer and Questioning Youth. Sponsored by OutProud, The National Coalition for Gay, Lesbian, Bisexual and Transgender Youth and *Oasis Magazine.* Contact survey@outproud.org.

Laan, E., Sonderman, M., & Janssen, E. (1996, June). Straight and lesbian women's sexual responses to straight and lesbian erotica: No sexual orientation effects. Paper presented at the annual meeting of the International Academy of Sex Research, Rotterdam, The Netherlands.

LaBarbera, P. (1994, February). Gay youth suicide: Myth is used to promote homosexual agenda. *Insight,* published by the Family Research Council; available at www.frc.org/insight/is94b3hs.html.

Larsson, I., & Svedin, C. G. (2002). Sexual experiences in childhood: Young adults' recollections. *Archives of Sexual Behavior, 31,* 263–273.

Laumann, E. O., Gagnon, J., Michael, R. T., & Michaels, S. (1994). *The social organization of sexuality: Sexual practices in the United States.* Chicago: University of Chicago Press.

Lebson, M. (2002). Suicide among homosexual youth. *Journal of Homosexuality, 42,* 107–117.

Levey, B. (2002, June 14). Gays at the prom: Less of an issue than ever. *Washington Post,* C11.

Levine, H. (1997). A further exploration of the lesbian identity development process and its measurement. *Journal of Homosexuality, 34,* 67–78.

Levine, J. (2002). *Harmful to minors: The perils of protecting children from sex.* Minneapolis: University of Minnesota Press.

Lewin, T. (2004, February 29). The gay rights movement, settled down. *New York Times,* p. 5.

Lippa, R. A. (2000). Gender-related traits in gay men, lesbian women, and heterosexual men and women: The virtual identity of homosexual-heterosexual diagnosticity and gender diagnosticity. *Journal of Personality, 68,* 899–926.

Lipsky, D. (1998, August 6). To be young and gay. *Rolling Stone,* pp. 55–65, 80, 82–85.

Lock, J., & Steiner, H. (1999a). Gay, lesbian, and bisexual youth risks for emotional, physical, and social problems: Results from a community-based survey. *Journal of the American Academy of Child and Adolescent Psychiatry, 38,* 297–304.

Lock, J., & Steiner, H. (1999b). Relationships between sexual orientation and coping styles of gay, lesbian, and bisexual adolescents from a community high school. *Journal of the Gay and Lesbian Medical Association, 3,* 77–82.

Luthar, S. S., Cicchetti, D., & Becker, B. (2000). The construct of resilience: A critical evaluation and guidelines for future work. *Child Development, 71,* 543–562.

Lynch, L. (2002, February 15–17). Questions. *USA Weekend,* p. 2.

Maccoby, E. E. (1998). *The two sexes: Growing up apart, coming together.* Cambridge, MA: Belknap Press of Harvard University Press.

Malyon, A. K. (1981). The homosexual adolescent: Developmental issues and social bias. *Child Welfare, 60,* 321–330.

Manalansan, M. F. (1996). Double minorities: Latino, Black, and Asian men who have sex with men. In R. C. Savin-Williams & K. M. Cohen (Eds.), *The lives of lesbians, gays, and bisexuals: Children to adults* (pp. 393–415). Fort Worth, TX: Harcourt Brace College Publishing.

Marcia, J. E. (1966). Development and validation of ego identity status. *Journal of Personality and Social Psychology, 3,* 551–558.

Marcia, J. E. (1994). The empirical sense of ego identity. In H. A. Bosma, T. L. G. Groafsma, H. D. Grotevant, & D. J. deLevita (Eds.), *Identity and development: An interactive approach* (pp. 67–80). London: Sage.

Marech, R. (2004, February 8). Nuances of gay identities reflected in new language: "Homosexual" is passé in a "boi's" life. *San Francisco Chronicle.* Retrieved from www.sfgate.com/cgi-bin/article.cgi?file.

Martin, A. D. (1982). Learning to hide: The socialization of the gay adolescent. In S. C. Feinstein, J. G. Looney, A. Z. Schwartzberg, & A. D. & J. Sorosky (Eds.), *Adolescent psychiatry: Developmental and clinical studies* (vol. 10) (pp. 52–65). Chicago: University of Chicago Press.

Martin, A. D., & Hetrick, E. S. (1988). The stigmatization of the gay and lesbian adolescent. *Journal of Homosexuality, 15,* 163–183.

McClintock, M. K., & Herdt, G. (1996). Rethinking puberty: The development of sexual attraction. *Current Directions in Psychological Science, 5,* 178–183.

McConaghy, N. (1999). Unresolved issues in scientific sexology. *Archives of Sexual Behavior, 28,* 285–318.

McConnell, J. H. (1994). Lesbian and gay male identities as paradigms. In S. L. Archer (Ed.), *Interventions for adolescent identity development* (pp. 103–118). Thousand Oaks, CA: Sage.

McDaniel, J. S., Purcell, D., & D'Augelli, A. R. (2001). The relationship between sexual orientation and risk for suicide: Research findings and future directions for research and prevention. *Suicide and Life-Threatening Behavior, 31* (Supplement), 84–105.

McDonald, G. J. (1982). Individual differences in the coming out process for gay men: Implications for theoretical models. *Journal of Homosexuality, 8,* 47–60.

McWhirter, D. P., Sanders, S. A., & Reinisch, J. M. (Eds.) (1990). *Homosexuality/heterosexuality: Concepts of sexual orientation.* New York: Oxford University Press.

Mead, M. (1970). *Culture and commitment: A study of the generation gap.* New York: Natural History Press.

Meyer, I. H. (2003). Prejudice, social stress, and mental health in lesbian, gay, and bisexual populations: Conceptual issues and research evidence. *Psychological Bulletin, 129,* 674–697.

Meyer-Bahlburg, H. F. L. (1984). Psychoendocrine research on sexual orientation: Current status and future options. *Progress in Brain Research, 61,* 375–398.

Miller, E. M. (2000). Homosexuality, birth order, and evolution: Toward an equilibrium reproductive economics of homosexuality. *Archives of Sexual Behavior, 29,* 1–34.

Minton, H. L., & McDonald, G. J. (1983–1984). Homosexual identity formation as a developmental process. *Journal of Homosexuality, 9,* 91–104.

Minzesheimer, B. (2000, September 14). "Listener" tells tales from Maupin's life. *USA Today,* pp. 1D–2D.

Mohr, J. J. (2002). Heterosexual identity and the heterosexual therapist: An identity perspective on sexual orientation dynamics in psychotherapy. *Counseling Psychologist, 30,* 532–566.

Molloy, M., & McLaren, S. (in press). Suicide? The right decision. The attitudes of heterosexual university students towards the suicide of gay, lesbian and heterosexual peers.

Moran, T. (2000, August 7). Mary Cheney's gay—so what? *USA Today.*

Morris, J. F. (1997). Lesbian coming out as a multidimensional process. *Journal of Homosexuality, 33,* 1–22.

Muehlenhard, C. L. (2000). Categories and sexuality. *Journal of Sex Research, 37,* 101–107.

Muehrer, P. (1995). Suicide and sexual orientation: A critical summary of recent research and directions for future research. *Suicide and Life-Threatening Behavior, 25* (Supplement), 72–81.

Mustanski, B. (2003). *Semantic heterogeneity in the definition of "having sex" for homosexuals.* Manuscript submitted for publication.

Mustanski, B. S., Chivers, M. L., & Bailey, J. M. (2002). A critical review of recent biological research on human sexual orientation. *Annual Review of Sex Research, 13,* 69–140.

Musto, M. (2004, March). Liz Phair. *Out,* p. 70.

New York Times. (2003, December 28). Year end review of music. Arts & Leisure, p. 32.

Nycum, B. (2000). *The XY survival guide: Everything you need to know about being young and gay.* San Francisco: XY Publishing.

Okami, P., Olmstead, R., & Abramson, P. R. (1997). Sexual experiences in early childhood: Eighteen-year longitudinal data from the UCLA family lifestyles project. *Journal of Sex Research, 34,* 339–347.

Orenstein, A. (2001). Substance use among gay and lesbian adolescents. *Journal of Homosexuality, 41,* 1–15.

Papadopoulos, N. G., Stamboulides, P., & Triantafillou, T. (2000). The psychosexual development and behavior of university students: A nationwide survey in Greece. *Journal of Psychology and Human Sexuality, 11,* 93–110.

Pattatucci, A. M. L., & Hamer, D. H. (1995). Development and familiality of sexual orientation in females. *Behavior Genetics, 25,* 407–420.

Peplau, L. A., & Garnets, L. D. (2000). A new paradigm for understanding women's sexuality. *Journal of Social Issues, 56,* 329–350.

Peplau, L. A., Garnets, L. D., Spalding, L. R., Conley, T. D., & Veniegas, R. C. (1998). A critique of Bem's "exotic becomes erotic" theory of sexual orientation. *Psychological Review, 105,* 387–394.

Peplau, L. A., Spalding, L. R., Conley, T. D., & Veniegas, R. C. (1999). The development of sexual orientation in women. *Annual Review of Sex Research, 10,* 70–99.

Peterson, J., & Bedogne, M. (Eds.) (2003). *A face in the crowd: Expressions of gay life in America.* Sparks, NV: Prospect Publishing.

Peterson, J. L., Folkman, S., & Bakeman, R. (1996). Stress, coping, HIV status, psychosocial resources, and depressive mood in African American, gay, bisexual, and heterosexual men. *American Journal of Community Psychology, 24,* 461–485.

Phillips, G., & Over, R. (1992). Adult sexual orientation in relation to memories of childhood gender conforming and gender nonconforming behaviors. *Archives of Sexual Behavior, 21,* 543–558.

Phillips, G., & Over, R. (1995). Differences between heterosexual, bisexual, and lesbian women in recalled childhood experiences. *Archives of Sexual Behavior, 24,* 1–20

Plummer, K. (1975). *Sexual stigma: An interactionist account.* Boston: Routledge & Kegan Paul.

Porter, D. (2001, December 7). Needs assessment survey study. Paper presented at the GLSEN Research Roundtable. www.apa.org/ed/hlgb.html.

Rahman, Q., & Wilson, G. D. (2003). Born gay? The psychobiology of human sexual orientation. *Personality and Individual Differences, 34,* 1337–82.

Regan, P. C., & Berscheid, E. (1995). Gender differences in beliefs about the causes of male and female sexual desire. *Personal Relationships, 2,* 345–358.

Remafedi, G. (1985). Adolescent homosexuality: Issues for pediatricians. *Clinical Pediatrics, 24,* 481–485.

Remafedi, G. (1987a). Male homosexuality: The adolescent's perspective. *Pediatrics, 79,* 326–330.

Remafedi, G. (1987b). Adolescent homosexuality: Psychosocial and medical implications. *Pediatrics, 79,* 331–337.

Remafedi, G. (1999a, October 6). Sexual orientation and youth suicide. *Journal of the American Medical Association, 282,* 1291–1292.

Remafedi, G. (1999b). Suicide and sexual orientation: Nearing the end of controversy? *Archives of General Psychiatry, 56,* 885–886.

Remafedi, G., French, S., Story, M., Resnick, M. D., & Blum, R. (1998). The relationship between suicide risk and sexual orientation: Results of a population-based study. *American Journal of Public Health, 88,* 57–60.

Remafedi, G., Resnick, M., Blum, R., & Harris, L. (1992). Demography of sexual orientation in adolescents. *Pediatrics, 89,* 714–721.

Reuters News Service (2001, March 14). More Americans having gay sex, study shows. Retrieved from www.reuters.com.

Reuters News Service (2003, May 27). Bravo to keep gay reality date. Retrieved from www.reuters.com.

Rind, B. (2001). Gay and bisexual adolescent boys' sexual experiences with men: An empirical examination of psychological correlates in a nonclinical sample. *Archives of Sexual Behavior, 30,* 345–368.

Robb, G. (2004). *Strangers: Homosexual love in the nineteenth century.* New York: W. W. Norton.

Rodríguez Rust, P. C. R. (2000). *Bisexuality in the United States: A social science reader.* New York: Columbia University Press.

Rodríguez Rust, P. C. (2001). Two many and not enough: The meanings of bisexual identities. *Journal of Bisexuality, 1,* 31–68.

Rodríguez Rust, P. C. R. (2002). Bisexuality: The state of the union. *Annual Review of Sex Research, 13,* 180–240.

Roesler, T., & Deisher, R. W. (1972, February 21). Youthful male homosexuality: Homosexual experience and the process of developing homosexual identity in males aged 16 to 22 years. *JAMA, 219(8),* 1018–1023.

Rosario, M., Meyer-Bahlburg, H. F. L., Hunter, J., Exner, T. M. Gwadz, M., & Keller, A. M. (1996). The psychosexual development of urban lesbian, gay, and bisexual youths. *Journal of Sex Research, 33,* 113–126.

Rosario, M., Meyer-Bahlburg, H. F. L., Hunter, J., & Gwadz, M. (1999). Sexual risk behaviors of gay, lesbian, and bisexual youths in New York City: Prevalence and correlates. *AIDS Education and Prevention, 11,* 476–496.

Rose, S. (2000). Heterosexism and the study of women's romantic and friend relationships. *Journal of Social Issues, 56,* 315–328.

Rothblum, E. D. (2000). Sexual orientation and sex in women's lives: Conceptual and methodological issues. *Journal of Social Issues, 56,* 193–204.

Rotheram-Borus, M. J., Hunter, J., & Rosario, M. (1994). Suicidal behavior and gay-related stress among gay and bisexual male adolescents. *Journal of Adolescent Research, 9,* 498–508.

Rotheram-Borus, M. J., Meyer-Bahlburg, H. F. L., Kooperman, C., Rosario, M., Exner, T. M., Henderson, R., Matthieu, M., & Gruen, R. S. (1992). Lifetime sexual behaviors among runaway males and females. *Journal of Sex Research, 29,* 15–29.

Rotheram-Borus, M. J., Rosario, M., Van Rossem, R., Reid, H., & Gillis, J. R. (1995). Prevalence, course, and predictors of multiple problem behaviors among gay and bisexual male adolescents. *Developmental Psychology, 31,* 75–85.

Ruoff, J. (2001). *An American family: A televised life.* Minneapolis: University of Minnesota Press.

Russell, G. M., Bohan, J. S., & Lilly, D. (2000). Queer youth: Old stories, new stories. In S. L. Jones (Ed.), *A sea of stories: The shaping power of narrative in gay and lesbian cultures* (pp. 69–92). New York: Harrington Park Press.

Russell, S. T., & Joyner, K. (2001). Adolescent sexual orientation and suicide risk: Evidence from a national study. *American Journal of Public Health, 91,* 1276–1281.

Russell, S. T., Seif, H., & Truong, N. L. (2001). School outcomes of sexual minority youth in the United States: Evidence from a national study. *Journal of Adolescence, 24,* 111–127.

Russell, S. T., & Truong, N. L. (2002, April). Adolescent sexual orientation, ethnicity, and school achievement. Paper presented at the ninth biennial meeting of the Society for Research on Adolescence, New Orleans, LA.

Rust, P. C. (1992). The politics of sexual identity: Sexual attraction and behavior among lesbian and bisexual women. *Social Problems, 39,* 366–386.

Rust, P. C. (1993). Coming out in the age of social constructionism: Sexual identity formation among lesbians and bisexual women. *Gender and Society, 7,* 50–77.

Rutter, M. (1987). Psychosocial resilience and protective mechanisms. *American Journal of Orthopsychiatry, 57,* 316–371.

Ryan, C. (2000, March 15). *An analysis of the content and gaps in the scientific and professional literature on the health and mental concerns of lesbian, gay and bisexual youth.* Paper prepared for the American Psychological Association Healthy LGB Students Project.

Saewyc, E. M., Skay, C. L., Bearinger, L. H., Blum, R. W., & Resnick, M. D. (1998). Demographics of sexual orientation among American Indian adolescents. *American Orthopsychiatric Association, 68,* 590–600.

Saghir, M. T., & Robbins, E. (1973). *Male and female homosexuality.* Baltimore, MD: Williams & Wilkins.

Sanders, S. A., & Reinisch, J. M. (1999). Would you say you "had sex" if . . . ? *Journal of the American Medical Association, 281,* 275–277.

Sandfort, T. G. M. (1992). The argument for adult-child sex: A critical appraisal and new data. In W. O'Donohue & J. H. Geer (Eds.), *The sexual abuse of children: Vol. 1, Theory and research* (pp. 38–48). Hillside, NJ: Erlbaum.

Sandfort, T. G. M. (1997). Sampling male homosexuality. In J. Bancroft (Ed.), *Researching sexual behavior: Methodological issues* (pp. 261–275). Bloomington: Indiana University Press.

Sandfort, T. G. M. (2003, July 19). Sexual orientation and gender: Stereotypes and beyond. Presidential address, 29th Annual Meeting of the International Academy of Sex Research, Bloomington, IN.

Savin-Williams, R. C. (1990). *Gay and lesbian youth: Expressions of identity.* Washington, DC: Hemisphere.

Savin-Williams, R. C. (1994). Verbal and physical abuse as stressors in the lives of sexual minority youth: Associations with school problems, running away, substance abuse, prostitution, and suicide. *Journal of Consulting and Clinical Psychology, 62,* 261–269.

Savin-Williams, R. C. (1995). An exploratory study of pubertal maturation timing and self-esteem among gay and bisexual male youths. *Developmental Psychology, 31,* 56–64.

Savin-Williams, R. C. (1996). Ethnic- and sexual-minority youth. In R. C. Savin-Williams & K. M. Cohen (Eds.), *The lives of lesbians, gays, and bisexuals: Children to adults.* (pp. 152–165). Fort Worth, TX: Harcourt Brace College Publishing.

Savin-Williams, R. C. (1998a). *". . . and then I became gay": Young men's stories.* New York: Routledge.

Savin-Williams, R. C. (1998b). The disclosure to families of same-sex attractions by lesbian, gay, and bisexual youths. *Journal of Research on Adolescence, 8,* 49–68.

Savin-Williams, R. C. (1999). Matthew Shepard's death: A professional awakening. *Applied Developmental Science, 3,* 150–154.

Savin-Williams, R. C. (2001a). A critique of research on sexual-minority youth. *Journal of Adolescence, 24,* 15–23.

Savin-Williams, R. C. (2001b). *"Mom, Dad, I'm gay": How families negotiate coming out.* Washington, DC: American Psychological Association.

Savin-Williams, R. C. (2001c). Suicide attempts among sexual-minority youth: Population and measurement issues. *Journal of Consulting and Clinical Psychology, 69,* 983–991.

Savin-Williams, R. C. (2003). Are adolescent same-sex romantic relationships on our radar screen? In P. Florsheim (Ed.), *Adolescent romantic relations and sexual behavior: Theory, research, and practical implications* (pp. 325–336). Mahwah, NJ: Lawrence Erlbaum.

Savin-Williams, R. C. (2004). Boy-on-boy sexuality. In N. Way & J. Y. Chu (Eds.), *Adolescent boys: Exploring diverse cultures of boyhood.* New York: New York University Press.

Savin-Williams, R. C. (in preparation). *". . . and then I kissed her": Young women's stories.*

Savin-Williams, R. C., & Diamond, L. M. (1997). Sexual orientation as a developmental context for lesbians, gays, and bisexuals: Biological perspectives. In N. L. Segal, G. E. Weisfeld, & C. C. Weisfeld (Eds.), *Uniting psychology and biology: Integrative perspectives on human development* (pp. 217–238). Washington, DC: American Psychological Association.

Savin-Williams, R. C., & Diamond, L. M. (1999). Sexual orientation. In

W. K. Silverman & T. H. Ollendick (Eds.), *Developmental issues in the clinical treatment of children* (pp. 241–258). Boston: Allyn & Bacon.

Savin-Williams, R. C., & Diamond, L. M. (2000). Sexual identity trajectories among sexual-minority youth: Gender comparisons. *Archives of Sexual Behavior, 29,* 419–440.

Savin-Williams, R. C., & Diamond, L. M. (2004). Sex. In R. M. Lerner & L. Steinberg (Eds.), *Handbook of adolescent psychology* (2nd ed.) (pp. 189–231). New York: John Wiley & Sons.

Savin-Williams, R. C., & Ream, G. L. (2003a). Sex variations in the disclosure to parents of same-sex attractions. *Journal of Family Psychology, 17,* 429–438.

Savin-Williams, R. C., & Ream, G. L. (2003b). Suicide attempts among sexual-minority male youth. *Journal of Clinical Child and Adolescent Psychology, 32,* 509–522.

Savin-Williams, R. C., & Ream, G. L. (in preparation–a). Stability and consistency of same-sex romantic attraction, sexual behavior, and sexual orientation identity in adolescence and young adulthood. Cornell University, Ithaca, NY.

Savin-Williams, R. C., & Ream, G. L. (in preparation–b). Age of puberty and sexual orientation in an adolescent national probability sample. Cornell University, Ithaca, NY.

Scalia, R. (2003, September 27). When roots, sexuality clash. *Montreal Gazette,* pp. E1–E3.

Scheufele, D. A. (2004, March 15). Gay marriage? Not this election. *Ithaca Journal,* p. 11A.

Schneider, M. (1989). Sappho was a right-on adolescent: Growing up lesbian. *Journal of Homosexuality, 17,* 111–130.

Schneider, M. S. (2001). Toward a reconceptualization of the coming-out process for adolescent females. In A. R. D'Augelli & C. J. Patterson (Eds.), *Lesbian, gay, and bisexual identities and youth: Psychological perspectives* (pp. 71–96). New York: Oxford University Press.

Schulman, S. (2004, January–February). What became of "freedom summer"? *Gay and Lesbian Review, 11,* pp. 20–21.

Schwarz, N. (1999). Self-reports: How the questions shape the answers. *American Psychologist, 54,* 93–105.

Sears, J. T. (1991). *Growing up gay in the South: Race, gender, and journeys of the spirit.* New York: Harrington Park Press.

Sell, R. L. (1996). The Sell Assessment of Sexual Orientation: Background and scoring. *Journal of Gay, Lesbian, and Bisexual Identity, 1,* 295–310.

Sell, R. L. (1997). Defining and measuring sexual orientation: A review. *Archives of Sexual Behavior, 26,* 643–658.

Sell, R. L., Wells, J. A., & Wypij, D. (1995). The prevalence of homosexual behavior and attraction in the United States, the United Kingdom, and France: Results of national population-based samples. *Archives of Sexual Behavior, 24,* 235–248.

Sengupta, S. (1999, November 6). By the way, a mayor-elect is gay. *New York Times,* B-5.

Shaffer, D., Fisher, P., Hicks, R. H., Parides, M., & Gould, M. (1995). Sexual orientation in adolescents who commit suicide. *Suicide and Life-Threatening Behavior, 35* (Supplement), 64–71.

Shaikin, B. (2000, September 18). Coming out to face the team. *Los Angeles Times.* Retrieved from newsdesk@channelq.com.

Sharp, D. (2003, December 8). Cities come out about wooing gays—and their dollars. *USA Today,* p. 3A.

Shively, M. G., & DeCecco, J. P. (1977). Components of sexual identity. *Journal of Homosexuality, 3,* 41–48.

Signorile, M. (1999, January 19). Ex-gay. Too gay. Postgay. What happened to gay? *The Advocate,* pp. 71, 73, 75, 77, 81.

Singh, D., Vidaurri, M., Zambarano, R. J., & Dabbs, J. M., Jr. (1999). Lesbian erotic role identification: Behavioral, morphological, and hormonal correlates. *Journal of Personality and Social Psychology, 76,* 1–15.

Smith, D. (2001, September). Assessing the needs of lesbian, gay, and bisexual youth. *Monitor on Psychology,* 42–43.

Smith-Rosenberg, C. (1985). *Disorderly conduct: Visions of gender in Victorian America.* New York: Alfred A. Knopf.

Sophie, J. (1985–1986). A critical examination of stage theories of lesbian identity development. *Journal of Homosexuality, 12,* 39–51.

Spence, J. T., & Helmreich, R. L. (1978). *Masculinity and femininity: Their psychological dimensions, correlates, and antecedents.* Austin: University of Texas Press.

Steinberg, L. (1995). Commentary: On developmental pathways and social contexts in adolescence, in L. J. Crockett & A. C. Crouter (Eds.), *Pathways through adolescence: Individual development in relation to social contexts,* pp. 245–253 (Mahwah, NJ: Lawrence Erlbaum).

Storms, M. D. (1981). A theory of erotic orientation development. *Psychological Review, 88,* 340–353.

Stukin, S. (2002, March 19). How the other half laughs. *The Advocate,* pp. 52–53.

Sullivan, H. S. (1953). *The interpersonal theory of psychiatry.* New York: W. W. Norton.

Suppe, F. (1984). In defense of a multidimensional approach to sexual identity. *Journal of Homosexuality, 10,* 7–14.

Sutton, M. J., Brown, J. D., Wilson, K. M., & Klein, J. D. (2002). Shaking the tree of knowledge for forbidden fruit: Where adolescents learn about sexuality and contraception. In J. D. Brown, J. R. Steele, & K. Walsh-Childers (Eds.), *Sexual teens, sexual media* (pp. 25–55). Mahwah, NJ: Erlbaum.

Szalacha, L. (2001). The sexual diversity climate of Massachusetts' secondary schools and the success of the Safe Schools Program for gay and lesbian students. Unpublished doctoral dissertation, Harvard University, Cambridge, MA.

Tannahill, R. (1980). *Sex in history.* New York: Stein and Day.

Tartagni, D. (1978). Counseling gays in a school setting. *School Counselor, 26,* 26–32.

Telljohann, S. K., & Price, J. H. (1993). A qualitative examination of adolescent homosexuals' life experiences: Ramifications for secondary school personnel. *Journal of Homosexuality, 26,* 41–56.

Terman, L. M., & Miles, C. C. (1936). *Sex and personality: Studies in masculinity and femininity.* New York: Russell & Russell.

Thompson, S. (1995). *Going all the way: Teenage girls' tales of sex, romance, and pregnancy.* New York: Hill and Wang.

Tofiño, I. (2003, May–June). Spain and the "Mediterranean model." *Gay and Lesbian Review, 10,* 17–18.

Tolman, D. L. (2002). *Dilemmas of desire: Teenage girls and sexuality.* Cambridge, MA: Harvard University Press.

Tolman, D. L., & Diamond, L. M. (2001). Desegregating sexuality research: Cultural and biological perspectives on gender and desire. *Annual Review of Sex Research, 12,* 33–74.

Troiden, R. R. (1979). Becoming homosexual: A model of gay identity acquisition. *Psychiatry, 42,* 362–373.

Troiden, R. R. (1984). Self, self-concept, identity, and homosexual identity: Constructs in need of definition and differentiation. *Journal of Homosexuality, 10,* 97–109.

Troiden, R. R. (1989). The formation of homosexual identities. *Journal of Homosexuality, 17,* 43–73.

Troiden, R. R., & Goode, E. (1980). Variables related to the acquisition of a gay identity. *Journal of Homosexuality, 5,* 383–392.

Udry, J. R., & Billy, J. O. G. (1987). Initiation of coitus in early adolescence. *American Sociological Review, 52,* 841–855.

Udry, J. R., Talbert, L. M., & Morris, N. M. (1986). Biosocial foundations for adolescent female sexuality. *Demography, 23,* 217–230.

Upchurch, D. M. (2002). Inconsistencies in reporting the occurrence and timing of first intercourse among adolescents. *Journal of Sex Research, 39,* 197–206.

Uribe, V., & Harbeck, K. M. (1991). Addressing the needs of lesbian, gay, and bisexual youth: The origins of PROJECT 10 and school-based intervention. *Journal of Homosexuality, 22,* 9–28.

USA Today (August 25, 2003). More companies adopt gay-friendly policies, report says. Retrieved from www.usatoday.com/money/companies.

Ward, L. M., & Rivadeneyra, R. (1999). Contributions of entertainment television to adolescents' sexual attitudes and expectations: The role of viewing amount versus viewer involvement. *Journal of Sex Research, 36,* 237–249.

Weeks, J. (1995). History, desire, and identities. In R. Parker & J. H. Gagnon (Eds.), *Conceiving sexuality: Approaches to sex research in a postmodern world* (pp. 33–50). London: Routledge.

Weinberg, M. S., Williams, C. J., & Pryor, D. W. (1994). *Dual attraction: Understanding bisexuality.* New York: Oxford University Press.

Weinberg, T. S. (1984). Biology, ideology, and the reification of developmental stages in the study of homosexual identities. *Journal of Homosexuality, 10,* 77–84.

Wheatcroft, G. (1999, August 30). Scouting for boys: The alternative lifestyle of Lord Baden-Powell, the first Boy Scout. *Slate Culture.*

Whoriskey, P. (2003, January 2). First D.C. baby of '03 has two moms. *Washington Post,* p. 10.

Wiederman, M. W. (1999). Volunteer bias in sexuality research using college student participants. *Journal of Sex Research, 36,* 59–66.

Williams, W. L. (1986). *The spirit and the flesh: Sexual diversity in American Indian culture.* Boston: Beacon Press.

Williams, W. L. (1996). Two-spirit persons: Gender nonconformity among Native American and Native Hawaiian youths. In R. C. Savin-Williams & K. M. Cohen (Eds.), *The lives of lesbians, gays, and bisexuals: Children to adults* (pp. 416–435). Fort Worth, TX: Harcourt Brace College Publishing.

Wloszczna, S. (2004, March 17). Affleck manages to laugh at life, love. Gannett News Service, *Ithaca Journal,* p. 8A.

Wooden, W. S., Kawasaki, H., & Mayeda, R. (1983). Lifestyles and identity maintenance among gay Japanese-American males. *Alternative Lifestyles, 5,* 236–243.

Worthington, R. L., Savoy, H. B., Dillon, F. R., & Vernaglia, E. R. (2002). Heterosexual identity development: A multidimensional model of individual and social identity. *Counseling Psychologist, 30,* 496–531.

Yang, A. S. (1997). Attitudes toward homosexuality. *Public Opinion Quarterly, 61,* 477–507.

Zacharek, S. (2003, August 3). An earlier Russell Crowe: The loving gay son. *New York Times,* p. 20.

Zernike, K. (2003, August, 24). The new couples next door, gay and straight. *New York Times,* p. 16.

Zucker, K. J. (Ed.) (2003, October). Special issue. *Archives of Sexual Behavior, 32*(5).

Index